T0295373

ERGOCHECK
for a Preliminary
Mapping of Risk at Work

Ergonomics Design and Management: Theory and Applications

Waldemar Karwowski

Industrial Engineering and Management Systems University of Central Florida (UCF) – Orlando, Florida

PUBLISHED TITLES

Risk Analysis and Management of Repetitive Actions

A Guide for Applying the OCRA System (Occupational Repetitive Actions),
Third Edition
Daniela Colombini and Enrico Occhipinti

Knowledge Service Engineering Handbook
Jussi Kantola and Waldemar Karwowski

Neuroadaptive Systems

Theory and Applications
*Magdalena Fafrowicz, Tadeusz Marek,
Waldemar Karwowski, and Dylan Schmorrow*

Safety Management in a Competitive Business Environment
Juraj Sinay

Ergonomics in Developing Regions

Needs and Applications
Patricia A. Scott

Human Factors of a Global Society

A System of Systems Perspective
*Tadeusz Marek, Waldemar Karwowski, Marek Frankowicz,
Jussi I. Kantola, and Pavel Zgaga*

Working Posture Assessment

The TACOS (Time-Based Assessment Computerized Strategy) Method
Daniela Colombini and Enrico Occhipinti

ERGOCHECK for a Preliminary Mapping of Risk at Work

Tools, Guidelines, and Applications
Daniela Colombini and Enrico Occhipinti

For more information about this series, please visit: https://www.crcpress.com/Ergonomics-Design--Mgmt-Theory--Applications/book-series/CRCEDMTAPPS

ERGOCHECK
for a Preliminary
Mapping of Risk at Work
Tools, Guidelines, and Applications

Edited by
Daniela Colombini and Enrico Occhipinti

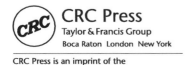

CRC Press
Taylor & Francis Group
Boca Raton London New York

CRC Press is an imprint of the
Taylor & Francis Group, an **informa** business

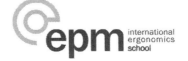

international
ergonomics
school

First edition published 2020
by CRC Press
6000 Broken Sound Parkway NW, Suite 300, Boca Raton, FL 33487-2742

and by CRC Press
2 Park Square, Milton Park, Abingdon, Oxon, OX14 4RN

© 2020 Taylor & Francis Group, LLC
CRC Press is an imprint of Taylor & Francis Group, LLC

Reasonable efforts have been made to publish reliable data and information, but the author and publisher cannot assume responsibility for the validity of all materials or the consequences of their use. The authors and publishers have attempted to trace the copyright holders of all material reproduced in this publication and apologize to copyright holders if permission to publish in this form has not been obtained. If any copyright material has not been acknowledged please write and let us know so we may rectify in any future reprint.

Except as permitted under U.S. Copyright Law, no part of this book may be reprinted, reproduced, transmitted, or utilized in any form by any electronic, mechanical, or other means, now known or hereafter invented, including photocopying, microfilming, and recording, or in any information storage or retrieval system, without written permission from the publishers.

For permission to photocopy or use material electronically from this work, access www.copyright. com or contact the Copyright Clearance Center, Inc. (CCC), 222 Rosewood Drive, Danvers, MA 01923, 978-750-8400. For works that are not available on CCC please contact mpkbookspermissions@ tandf.co.uk

Trademark notice: Product or corporate names may be trademarks or registered trademarks, and are used only for identification and explanation without intent to infringe.

Library of Congress Cataloging-in-Publication Data
Names: Colombini, Daniela, editor. | Occhipinti, Enrico, editor.
Title: ERGOCHECK, for a preliminary mapping of risk at work: tools, guidelines, and applications / edited by Daniela Colombini and Enrico Occhipinti.
Other titles: ERGOCHECK, un metodo per la mappatura preliminare dei fattori di rischio per la salute e il benessere al lavoro. English
Description: Boca Raton, FL: CRC Press, 2020. | Series: Ergonomics design & mgmt. theory & applications | "This book was previously published in Italian entitled, 'ERGOCHECK un metodo per la mappatura preliminare dei fattori di rischio per la salute e il benessere al lavoro. Strumento, modalità di uso, esempi applicative.' By Daniela Colombini, Enrico Occhipinti No 1125, 2019; published by Dossier Ambiente, Milano, Italy." | Includes bibliographical references and index.
Identifiers: LCCN 2019056387 | ISBN 9780367230098 (hardback) | ISBN 9780429281556 (ebook)
Subjects: LCSH: Industrial safety–Data processing. | Industrial hygiene–Data processing. | Work environment–Case studies–Data processing. | Risk assessment–Data processing. | Employees–Health risk assessment–Data processing. | Lists–Data processing. | ErgoCheck.
Classification: LCC T55.3.D38 E74 2020 | DDC 658.3/820285–dc23

ISBN: 978-0-367-23009-8 (hbk)
ISBN: 978-0-429-28155-6 (ebk)

Typeset in Times
by codeMantra

This book was previously published in Italian entitled, "ERGOCHECK un metodo per la mappatura preliminare dei fattori di rischio per la salute e il benessere al lavoro. Strumento, modalità di uso, esempi applicative. By Daniela Colombini, Enrico Occhipinti

No 1125, 2019; published by Dossier Ambiente, Milano, Italy.

We have fond memories of when, as recent graduates in occupational medicine, we were sent by Prof. Antonio Grieco and Prof. Giulio Maccacaro to a factory to evaluate the health problems of the "working class". There were no tools back then other than talking with workers, listening to their problems and reporting "worker subjectivity through homogeneous groups". This was back in 1974–1975. We knew precious little about occupational health "in the field" but were fast learners and soon found simple ways of detecting the preventive needs of workers and their priorities. We dedicate this volume, which emphasizes the need to focus on subjectivity through the use of simple guidelines and evaluation tools, to our mentors Prof. Antonio Grieco and Prof. Giulio Maccacaro.

THE HOMOGENEOUS WORKER GROUP, GENERATING KNOWLEDGE THROUGH COLLECTIVE SUBJECTIVITY (Giulio Maccacaro, 1970s)

It is through this process and with this outlook that the Italian workers' movement in 1968 became aware that the traditional approach, based on the "neutrality", "objectivity", and "uniqueness" of the production cycle and of the technology and science driving it, is no longer acceptable. There is no point in acquiring an abstract snapshot of the production process; what is needed is a real depiction of what each member of the working group experiences as his or her own personal condition. Of course, this depiction is not an individualistic view but rather the result of an evaluation and exploration of the different individualities that contribute, each with their own subjectivity, to constituting the Homogeneous Worker Group and their collective subjectivity. To achieve this, it is necessary to understand how the work of the Homogeneous Worker Group is actually organized and how the group experiences it, together with their working and social backgrounds and real working conditions.

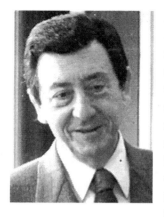

ANTONIO GRIECO is a distinguished Teacher and Researcher, a Mentor to all those involved in Prevention, and for over 15 years, the Director of the "Clinica del Lavoro-Luigi Devoto" at the University of Milan. His contribution to the development of Occupational Medicine at the national and international levels and his political and social commitments have profoundly shaped the development of the discipline over the last 40 years and significantly enhanced prevention and the protection of workers' health. He was one of the first Italian experts in ergonomics. He founded (together with other colleagues)

- the Italian Society of Ergonomics (1969);
- EPM, the Research Unit of Ergonomics of
Posture and Movement (1985);
- CIIP, the Italian Inter-associative Council for Prevention (1990).

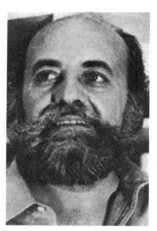

GIULIO ALFREDO MACCACARO is a prominent physician and academic since 1964. He taught medical statistics and biometrics at the University of Milan. And as an advocate of scientific dissent, he spearheaded a movement calling for the renewal, on a democratic basis, of the organization of health care in Italy (Democratic Medicine) and fought against human experimentation and drug consumerism.

Contents

Preface

In recent years, there has been an undeniable increase in the number of complex, multifactorial work-related disorders and diseases in the working population. Only a "holistic" approach can hope to prevent these work-related health effects such as musculoskeletal disorders (WMSDs) and other issues generated by occupational stress. National and international prevention agencies and professionals are therefore searching for simple tools that they can use for assessing and managing specific work-related risk factors, but that non-experts can also employ in both developed and developing countries, especially in very small businesses, small and medium enterprises (SMEs), and non-industrial sectors.

For years now, the World Health Organization (WHO) has encouraged the development of "toolkits" to make it easier to identify occupational risks and disorders. In describing how such a toolkit should be designed, the WHO indicates a set of practical risk assessment procedures and guidelines, including advice on simple risk control options (WHO, 2010). The toolkit should thus be simple and easy to use even by non-specialists in SMEs and developing countries.

The Milan-based International School of Ergonomics of Posture and Movements (EPMIES) has played an active role in designing a toolkit for analyzing and managing the risks associated with biomechanical overload and preventing WMSDs, in cooperation with the WHO and the International Ergonomics Association (IEA), along with other agencies operating under the International Organization for Standardization (ISO) and International Labour Office (ILO).

Much space within this project is obviously allocated to defining simple risk factor analysis tools that can also be used by non-experts in ergonomics, occupational health or industrial hygiene.

Acknowledgement

We thank Dr. Elena Guerrera, Dr. Marina Mameli and Dr. Daniela Sarto for the decisive contribution provided in the validation of the chapters dedicated to the bio-risk pre-mapping in this book and in ERGOCHECK software.

Editors

Sergio Ardissone was a Coordinator at the ASL Asti Prevention and Safety Service from 1974 to 2014. He followed the training course "The prevention and risk management of musculoskeletal biomechanical overload of the upper limbs and spine" organized by EPM Research Unit Ergonomics of posture and movement in Milan. He has a long professional experience in assessing the risk of biomechanical overload. He is the author or co-author of scientific publications on the topics, prevenction of professional biomechanical overload and accredited teacher of the EPM International Ergonomic School. s.ardissone@tin.it

Alberto Baratti earned his graduation in medicine and surgery, specialization in occupational medicine, and master's degree in pulmonology and respiratory physiopathology. Since 1988, he has worked in territorial and hospital occupational health services. In 2003, he was the Director at the ASL CN 1and in 2018 at the ASO S. Croce and Carle di Cuneo. Since 1989, he has delivered talks at conferences and taught regional and national training courses. He was an Adjunct Professor of ergonomics for the 3-year degree course of TPALL at the University of Turin (2010–2011) and, from 2015 to date, of occupational medicine for a degree course in work psychology. Since 2004, he has been responsible for several projects of the Piemonte Region on the promotion of health and safety in health facilities, in particular for ergonomics, work-related stress and safety management systems (SGSL). He has participated in various national working groups on ergonomics, in particular EPMIES (Member and Professor of the EPMIES scientific association), SIMLII and Coordination of Regions, and on work-related stress. albertobaratti60@gmail.com

Paolo Campanini earned his Ph.D. in occupational medicine. He is a Work and Organization Psychologist and Psychotherapist. He worked in the Clinica del Lavoro of Milan. As a former research fellow at the University of Milan, he has written scientific papers published in national and international scientific journals concerning work stress resulting from assessments, interventions and research carried out for national and multinational companies. He continues to work with interventions, training, assessments and research on psychosocial issues (such as engagement, well-being, work-related stress, mobbing and burnout) in multinational organizations. He has been a member and Professor of the EPMIES Scientific Association. www.paolocampanini.it

Ugo Caselli graduated in biological sciences and natural sciences, with specialization in biochemistry and clinical chemistry. From 1993 to 2000, he worked at the Neurobiology of Aging Center of the Research Department "N. Masera" of the INRCA (National Institute of Rest and Care for the Elderly) of Ancona, dealing with alterations in the nervous system, following the aging processes. Since 2001, he has been a Biologist at INAIL and dealt with issues concerning health and safety at work, in particular biological and ergonomic risks.

Daniela Colombini has a degree in medicine with postgraduate specialization in occupational medicine and health statistics. She is a certified European Ergonomist and a senior researcher at the Research Unit Ergonomics of Posture and Movement, Milan, where she developed methods for the analysis, evaluation and management of risk and damage from occupational biomechanical overload. She was a Professor at the School of Specialization in Occupational Medicine at the University of Milan and the University of Florence. She is the co-author of the *OCRA Method* (EN 1005-5 standard and ISO 11228-3). She is the Founder and President of the EPM International Ergonomics School EPMIES. She has been working with accredited native teachers in different countries such as USA, France, India, Spain, Chile, Colombia, Guatemala, Costa Rica, Brazil and other South American countries. She is a member of the Ergonomics Committee of UNI working in the international commissions of CEN and ISO. She is coordinator of a sub-group of Technical Committee on the Prevention of Musculoskeletal Disorders of the IEA. She has devoted more than 30 years on ergonomic issues related to physical ergonomics and the prevention of work-related musculoskeletal disorders, and is the author of more than 200 papers and handbooks, in Italian and English, on the matter. epmies.corsi@gmail.com, www.epmresearch.org

Giuseppina Coppola is a Surgeon and Occupational Medicine Specialist. From 2005 to 2007, she was a Volunteer Doctor at the University of Siena Rheumatology. In 2010, she collaborated with the EPM in the first applications of risk prematting with ERGOCHECK in small- and medium-sized enterprises. From November 2011 to the present, she is a Competent Physician at Tuscan companies of small and medium enterprises and, from 2016, Occupational Medical Doctor at the University of Siena. giuseppina_coppola@libero.it

Giorgio Di Leone is the Director of Occupational Prevention and Safety Service (SPESAL) North ASL Area BA, Technical Assistant in the Department of Health Policies of the Puglia Region, "National table" coordinator for the prevention of musculoskeletal system diseases, and Scientific Coordinator for Regional Targeted Plan "Risk Management by Manual Handling Patients in the Puglia Region" (MAPO). He is a Scientific Coordinator of the regional project "Prevention of osteoarticular pathologies related work in agriculture" and a Scientific Coordinator of the Ministry of Health for the purpose of research "Prevention of repetitive movements in workers in the upholstered furniture sector". g.dileone@tin.it

Maurizia Giambartolomei earned her degrees in medicine and surgery at the University of Bologna. Her specializations are in hygiene and preventive medicine and in occupational health at the University of Ancona. She carried out her professional activities mainly in Regione Marche (Ancona and neighboring towns), operating within the Prevention Department. She gained professional and managerial experience in occupational and public health by dealing with those issues characterizing this industrial area such as high-risk industrial plants (e.g. oil refinery), as well as a strong presence of maritime/port activities and shipbuilding industry.

While collaborating with public bodies and national institutions, she took part in various epidemiological studies and risk assessment researches regarding ergonomics, occupational health, work management, hygiene and safety in specific working fields such as fishery and the shipbuilding industry. mg@maume.it

Enrico Occhipinti has a degree in medicine with postgraduate specialization in occupational medicine and health statistics at the University of Milano (Italy). He is a Certified European Ergonomist. He is a Professor at the School of Specialization at the Occupational Medicine, University of Milan, and the Director of the Research Unit Ergonomics of Posture and Movement (EPM) at Fondazione Don Gnocchi ONLUS-Milano. He has devoted more than 30 years on ergonomic issues related to physical ergonomics and the prevention of work-related musculoskeletal disorders, and is the author of more than 250 papers and handbooks, in Italian and English, on the matter. He developed and co-authored the OCRA method. He is a member and has been a Coordinator of the Technical Committee on Prevention of Musculoskeletal Disorders of the International Ergonomics Association (IEA) and represents Italy in international commissions of the European Committee for Normalization (CEN) and the International Organization for Standardization (ISO) dealing with ergonomics and biomechanics.

Contributors

Sergio Ardissone
Professor, Ergonomics of Posture and
Movements International
Ergonomics School (EPM-IES)
Asti, Italy

Alberto Baratti
Director, Territorial and hospital
occupational medicine services
at ASL CN 1
Cuneo, Italy
and
Ergonomics of Posture and Movements
International Ergonomics School
(EPM-IES)
Milano, Italy

Paolo Campanini
Ergonomics of Posture and Movements
International Ergonomics School
(EPM-IES)
Milano, Italy

Ugo Caselli
l'INAIL
Ancona, Italy

Daniela Colombini
Ergonomics of Posture and Movements
International Ergonomics School
(EPM-IES)
Milano, Italy

Giuseppina Coppola
Rheumatology of the University of Siena
Siena, Italy

Giorgio Di Leone
Director, Workplace Prevention and
Safety Service (SPESAL) Area Nord
ASL BA
Bari, Italy

Maurizia Giambartolomei
Ancona, Italy

Loretta Montomoli
Rheumatology of the University of Siena
Siena, Italy

Enrico Occhipinti
Ergonomics of Posture and Movements
International Ergonomics School
(EPM-IES)
Milano, Italy

1 Introduction and Aim

Daniela Colombini and Enrico Occhipinti
Ergonomics of Posture and Movements
International Ergonomics School (EPM-IES)

In 2011, Ergonomics of Posture and Movements International Ergonomics School (EPMIES) began developing and fine-tuning a tool called ERGOCHECK that also took the latest international technical standards and field applications into account (Colombini and Occhipinti, 2011). The tool (and the relative software) was designed to recognize and provide a preliminary framework for the leading occupational risk factors (starting with biomechanical overload) affecting the health and wellbeing of workers.

The tool is part of a general occupational risk analysis and management model based on two main principles (Occhipinti and Colombini, 2016):

a. A step-by-step approach, starting with basic tools and gradually moving to more complex ones only when required for the purposes of prevention;
b. An awareness of every aspect of the numerous risk factors encountered at every step (albeit explored in different levels of detail).

With reference to the first principle, it is a well-known fact that the ISO technical standards adopt a general approach towards assessing and managing risk, following four fundamental steps: hazard/problem identification, simplified risk estimation, detailed risk evaluation and risk reduction.

With reference to the second principle, it goes without saying that at least in the initial mapping phase, all the principal risk factors for on-the-job health and welfare, from the ergonomic, occupational health and industrial hygiene standpoint, must be considered (i.e. biomechanical overload, noise, lighting, microclimate, vibrations, chemical and physical pollutants, work-related stress, etc.).

Figure 1.1 summarizes the levels of analysis suggested by the general model:

- **First level:** Preliminary identification of the main hazards (or issues) related to working conditions and priority setting through a series of "key questions" (or "key enters"). The focus here is on all potential hazards (or problems) with regard to ergonomics, industrial hygiene and occupational medicine. This level of analysis can be handled by non-specialists with limited training.
- **Second level:** This level involves performing a "Quick Assessment". Non-specialists with at least some basic training can handle this level of analysis.

1

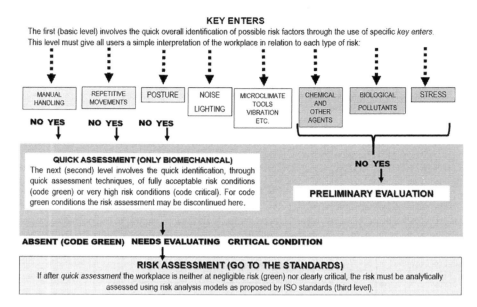

FIGURE 1.1   Levels of intervention for the identification, Quick Assessment and analysis of work-related risks.

- **Third level:** Based on the results of the second-level enquiry, risk is estimated using tools recognized by international standards and guidelines or published in the international literature. These tools must be capable of identifying the main risk factors. Only specialists with adequate training should conduct third-level assessments.

In this book, ERGOCHECK takes the general model shown in Figure 1.1 and focuses on the first two steps (i.e. identification and simplified assessment of potential risk factors), referring the reader to other sources for the more in-depth analytical steps.

ERGOCHECK was developed taking into account the following basic criteria:

- **Globality:** A global approach towards assessing the worker's discomfort, due to either the task, the workplace or the work organization.
- **Simplicity:** The easy-to-use methodology consists of a model for collecting data through interviews with workers but without specific measurements. The descriptive phase is comprised of closed-ended questions that are already provided by a devoted software.
- **Scale of priorities:** The results generated automatically by the software and depicted clearly in bar graphs not only help to identify problems but also offer a scale of priorities for putting in place subsequent risk assessment or risk reduction measures.
- **Involvement of the workers:** Worker involvement is critical for collecting information regarding the various risk factors (without adopting any measures) and assessing situations.

TABLE 1.1

Physical Risk Factors: Proportion (%) of EU-28 Workers Exposed to Various Physical Risk Factors for at Least 25% of Their Working Time (2005–2015)

	2005	2010	2015
Vibrations from handheld tools or machines	24	23	20
Noise loud enough to require raising the voice	30	29	28
High temperatures	25	22	23
Low indoor and outdoor temperatures	22	23	21
Breathing in fumes and/or dust	19	17	15
Breathing in vapors such as solvents	11	10	11
Handling or touching chemicals	14	15	17
Handling or being in direct contact with potentially infected materials	9	11	13
Tiring working postures	46	46	43
Lifting or moving people	8	9	10
Lifting or moving heavy loads	35	34	32
Repetitive hand or arm movements	62	63	61

Source: Eurofound (2017).

With regard to the first aspect (globality), it should be noted that all potential risk factors and causes of discomfort for the health and wellbeing of workers have been considered, while risks relating more closely to "traditional" industrial safety (accidents) have been deliberately excluded.

The authors have decided to leverage their extensive expertise and focus on aspects pertaining to biomechanical overload (also given the presence of specific international standards such as ISO/TR 12295 (ISO, 2014), which reflects the methodology adopted) and work-related stress, which represent the most widespread exposure conditions, at least among European workers, as can partly be inferred from Table 1.1 that derives from the 6th European Working Conditions Survey conducted in 2015 in all 28 EU countries (Eurofound, 2017).

For all the other factors, the work illustrated here represents the state of the art at the time of writing; however, it is reasonable to assume that this proposal will be amended over time, as regards both the factors considered and the way in which they are analyzed, provided that the simplification criteria underlying the proposal are maintained.

As to the third criterion (scale of priorities), it should be noted that the proposed methodology and software tool represent an initial systematic method for screening potential risks and causes of discomfort for human health, which cannot, however, be regarded as exhaustive for a comprehensive risk assessment, as required by international regulations, standards and guidelines. The aim is rather to examine workplaces and determine the main occupational risk factors that an in-depth assessment will subsequently need to focus on, or that require the adoption of measures to reduce risks and related consequences.

The tool is primarily designed to be used by employers and Health, Safety, and Environment/Prevention and Protection Services. It may also be used by occupational health physicians for periodical on-site inspections and for drafting health surveillance protocols, as well as by trade union representatives to periodically monitor hazardous situations in the workplace. Regulators may also find the software tool useful for conducting inspections in the workplace, to rapidly detect potentially dangerous situations requiring specific preventive interventions. This publication is in fact designed to assist the aforesaid professionals and operators.

The main features of the proposed methodology and software tool can be summarized as follows (Figure 1.1):

- The tool is based on the WHO's model of Key Questions, Quick Assessments and more in-depth investigations (only when necessary), which, with regard to biomechanical overload, are covered by ISO Technical Report 12295 (ISO, 2014).
- The tool takes into account all potential factors of risk and discomfort for human health (i.e. noise, lighting, microclimate, vibrations, machinery, biological agents, work-related stress, etc.) in addition to those deriving from biomechanical overload.
- For the main risk factors of biomechanical overload (as well as for pollutants and biological agents), a clear distinction is made between the Key-Enters phase and the Quick Assessment phase. For work-related stress there is just one Quick Assessment work sheet, as it is impossible to determine a single Key-Enter. For all the other factors, the two phases are intertwined.
- In all cases, the analysis is based exclusively on observational data (with no instrumental or other forms of measurement) and on a discussion with the *homogeneous group* of workers under study. Here *homogeneous group* refers to a group of workers performing the same task or set of tasks in the same workplace, for the same duration and with the same exposure conditions.
- In the case of biomechanical overload risk factors, the Quick Assessment phase not only generates "Definitely acceptable" and "Definitely critical" conditions, as per ISO/TR 12295, but also roughly estimates the priority level of the intermediate conditions, based on the approximations produced by the simple assessment tools proposed by ISO 11228 (parts 1, 2 and 3), (ISO, 2003, 2007a, 2007b).
- For pollutants, particularly chemical pollutants, a still rough but original approach was adopted to classify intervention priorities according to "control banding" models and criteria.
- In all cases and for all the aspects taken into consideration, the outcomes produced by the tool indicate the priority of attention (for a detailed, possibly instrumental assessment, or for intervention) for each of the risk factors considered: in other words, a preliminary approach that obviously cannot replace an in-depth assessment, but that does provide a useful indication of what to tackle first in terms of analyzing the current situation and perhaps adopting preventive measures.

2 Reference Sources

CONTENTS

2.1 REFERENCE SOURCES FOR STUDYING BIOMECHANICAL OVERLOAD: KEY ENTERS AND QUICK ASSESSMENT IN ISO/TR 12295

Daniela Colombini and Enrico Occhipinti
Ergonomics of Posture and Movements International Ergonomics School (EPM-IES)

Between the years 2000 and 2007, ISO published a series of technical standards on the physical ergonomics of working postures, manual handling (lifting, carrying, pushing and pulling) and repetitive manual tasks (ISO 11226 and series ISO 11228). Then in April 2014, a special application document was released (ISO/TR 12295) to better clarify the application modalities and procedures of the methods reported in these standards (ISO, 2000, 2003, 2007a, 2007 b, 2014).

The Technical Report addresses two main groups of users (non-experts and experts) to whom it devotes two separate sections:

- **The main text,** focussing on the identification of risk through Key Enters (field of application of the various standards in the series) and Quick Assessment.
- **A series of three annexes,** focussing on the three main parts of ISO 11228, with methodological insights into the methods used and with particular attention to the analysis of multiple tasks. No in-depth analysis has been conducted with regard to standard ISO 11226 on working postures, since there was insufficient application experience in the field.

It is worth pointing out that for ISO, a Technical Report is a sort of guideline describing the *state of the art* on a specific subject for which an actual standard has not yet been defined. Technical Reports generally provide only guidance and information. ISO/TR 12296 is a case in point, with reference to manual handling (of people) in the health-care sector.

ISO/TR 12295 is somewhat of a departure from the usual Technical Report, insofar as it describes the application of existing regulations and standards and simply broadens their scope and application but without amending the basic content and criteria (which in any case can only be done if the regulations are changed).

In Italy, since ISO/TR 12295 refers to the implementation of international standards expressly mentioned in Legislative Decree 81/08, it provides strict, valid and useful indications for the initial classification of the risk of biomechanical overload. In this respect, ISO/TR 12295 has been transposed and embedded into the guidelines recently issued by the Lombardy Region and also the guidelines produced by the Technical Coordination of the Italian Regions.

Only the parts of ISO/TR 12295 relating to Key Enters and Quick Assessment that will then become part of the more general ERGOCHECK tool will be reported here.

2.1.1 KEY ENTERS

Specific *Key Enters* are used to verify the existence of an occupational hazard or problem (*hazard identification*), in this case due to biomechanical overload and for Work-related Musculo-Skeletal Disorders (WMSDs), and to determine whether further analysis and evaluation are required.

Key Enters in fact define the scope of application of the four parts making up the relevant ISO standards.

Figure 2.1 shows the list of *key-enters* mentioned in ISO/TR 12295.

It should be noted that the only reason for indicating the presence of a situation (e.g., lifting a load of 3 kg or more; presence of a manual repetitive task) is to establish that it must be assessed; it does not suggest that there is necessarily any risk. The existence of risk will be established only after the next stage of the evaluation. Conversely, if there are no situations such as those described, then no further assessments are required.

1 Application of ISO 11228-1		
Is there manual lifting/lowering or carrying of an object of 3 kg or more present?	NO	YES
if **NO**, then this standard is not relevant, go to the next "Key Questions" regarding the other standards If **YES** then go to step 2 " Quick Assessment"		
2 Application of ISO 11228-2		
Is there a two-handed whole-body pushing and pulling of loads present?	NO	YES
if **NO**, then this standard is not relevant, go to the next "Key Questions" regarding the other standards If **YES** then go to step 2 "Quick Assessment"		
3 Application of ISO 11228-3		
Are there one or more repetitive tasks of the upper limbs with a total duration of 1 hour or more per shift? Where the definition of "repetitive task" is: *a task characterized by repeated work cycles* *or* *tasks during which the same working actions are repeated for more than 50% of the cycle time.*	NO	YES
If **NO**, then this standard is not relevant, go to the next "Key Questions" regarding the other standards If **YES** then go to step 2 "Quick Assessment"		
4 Application of ISO 11226		
Are there static or awkward working postures of the HEAD/NECK, TRUNK and/or UPPER AND LOWER LIMBS maintained for more than 4 seconds consecutively and repeated for a significant part of the working time? **For example:** - *HEAD/NECK (neck bent back/forward/sideways, twisted)* - *TRUNK (trunk bent forward/sideways/, bent back with no support, twisted)* - *UPPER LIMBS (hand(s) at or above head, elbow(s) at or above shoulder, elbow/hand(s) behind the body, hand(s) turned with palms completely up or down, extreme elbow flexion-extension, wrist bent forward/back/sideways)* - *LOWER LIMBS (squatting or kneeling) maintained for more than 4 seconds consecutively and repeated for a significant part of the working time*	NO	YES
if **NO**, then this standard is not relevant If **YES** then go to step 2 "Quick Assessment"		

FIGURE 2.1 ISO/TR 12295: Key Enters for the application of standards ISO 11226 and 11228 (parts 1-2-3).

2.1.2 QUICK ASSESSMENT

Quick Assessment is designed to make a rapid evaluation of any potential risks (e.g., manual load handling) by answering a set of simple qualitative and quantitative questions. Its purpose is essentially to simply detect three possible conditions (outputs):

- Acceptable (green): No further actions are required.
- Critical (purple): The work or process needs urgent redesigning.
- **A more detailed analysis is required:** An in-depth assessment is necessary using more detailed analytical tools (as suggested in this case by ISO 11228, parts 1, 2 and 3), which in turn may classify risk as acceptable (green), borderline (yellow) or present (red).

It is worth remembering that when conditions are found to be acceptable or critical, respectively, it is not always necessary to conduct a more in-depth analysis of the exposure level (second level), especially in the case of critical conditions. Efforts should be directed towards reducing the detected risk rather than on conducting often complex and sometimes useless investigations into the situation.

On the other hand, as happens in the majority of cases, if neither of these two "extreme" conditions are clearly detected, it is essential to assess risk using either a simplified or a more detailed approach and traditional assessment methods (such as those found in ISO/TR 12295). This assessment may result in risk being classified as green, yellow or red, with all the relevant operational consequences.

With reference to the recommendations set out in ISO/TR 12295 relating to tasks with Manual Handling of Loads (MHL) and ISO 11228 parts 1 and 2 (lifting and carrying, pushing and pulling), it should be noted that in both cases, the adequacy of certain settings must be first verified, as also mentioned in Annexes of the European Directive 269/90.

Figure 2.2 shows the preliminary conditions that must be examined with regard to manual *lifting and carrying*. It is important to note that if one or more of these preliminary conditions are inadequate, it cannot be established if the condition is fully acceptable or not, and steps must be taken to amend the inadequate conditions.

Is the working environment unfavourable for manual lifting and carrying?		
Presence of extreme (low or high) temperature	NO	YES
Presence of slippery, uneven, unstable floor	NO	YES
Presence of insufficient space for lifting and carrying	NO	YES
Are there unfavourable object characteristics for manual lifting and carrying?		
The size of object reduces the operator's view and hinder movement	NO	YES
The centre of gravity of the load is not stable (example: liquids, items moving around inside of object)	NO	YES
The object shape/configuration presents sharp edges, surfaces or protrusions	NO	YES
The contact surfaces are too cold or too hot	NO	YES
Does the task(s) with manual lifting or carrying last more than 8 hours a day?	NO	YES
If all of the questions are answered" NO", then continue the "Quick Assessment". If at least one of the questions is answered "YES", then APPLY The standard ISO 11228-1. The consequent specific additional risks HAVE TO be carefully considered to MINIMIZE THESE RISKS.		

FIGURE 2.2   Lifting and carrying: preliminary aspects.

LIFTING/LOWERING - Quick Assessment - Acceptable condition

		NO	YES
3 TO 5 kg	Asymmetry (e.g. body rotation, trunk twisting) is absent	NO	YES
	Load is maintained close to the body	NO	YES
	Load vertical displacement is between hips and shoulders	NO	YES
	Maximum frequency: less than 5 lifts per minute	NO	YES
5,1 TO 10 kg	Asymmetry (e.g. body rotation, trunk twisting) is absent	NO	YES
	Load is maintained close to the body	NO	YES
	Load vertical displacement is between hips and shoulder	NO	YES
	Maximum frequency: less than 1 lift per minute	NO	YES
MORE THAN 10 kg	Loads of more than 10 kg are absent	NO	YES

If all of the questions are answered "YES",
then the examined task is in green area (ACCEPTABLE) and it is not necessary to continue the risk evaluation.
If at least one of the questions is answered "NO", then evaluate the task(s) by ISO 11228-1.

Carrying - Quick Assessment - Acceptable condition

Recommended Cumulative Mass (total load (in kg) carried during the given durations for the specified distance below): is the cumulative mass carried LESS than recommended values considering the distance (more/less than 10 meters) and duration (1 minute; 1 hour; 8 hours)?

Duration	Distance ≤ 10 m per action	Distance > 10 m per action		
8 hrs	10000 kg	6000 kg	NO	YES
1 h	1500 kg	750 kg	NO	YES
1 min	30 kg	15 kg	NO	YES
	Awkward postures during the carrying are not present		NO	YES

If all of the questions are answered "YES",
then the examined task is in green area (ACCEPTABLE) and it is not necessary to continue the risk evaluation.
If at least one of the questions is answered "NO", then evaluate the task(s) by ISO 11228-1.

FIGURE 2.3 Lifting and carrying: Quick Assessment – acceptable conditions.

Moving on to acceptable conditions for lifting and carrying, Figure 2.3 shows a list of conditions that must *all be present simultaneously* in order to determine that the situation is acceptable (green). It should be noted that when conditions are defined as acceptable, they are deemed acceptable for the *healthy working population*, and not to specific individual health issues.

Figure 2.4 shows the potential critical conditions; in this case, when even just one condition is present, the situation is defined as *critical.*

To make a Quick Assessment of "*definitely critical*" conditions, reference has been made to the definitions and criteria included in the methods recommended by the standards (starting with the Revised National Institute for Occupational Safety and Health (NIOSH) Lifting Equation), which indicate one or more highly risky elements. These might include situations in which the parameters (multipliers) of the NIOSH equation are essentially equal to Ø or where the loads are heavier than the maximum weights recommended by standard ISO 11228-1.

If a manual handling condition is critical, even in just one of the situations listed in Figure 2.4, the recommendation is to opt immediately for rapid and substantial remedial actions (risk reduction) without necessarily conducting a more in-depth analytical evaluation, which can, however, be carried out at a later stage to verify the potential effectiveness of the corrective measures put in place.

Also, as regards the Quick Assessment of whole-body *pushing and pulling*, several significant preliminary aspects must be examined.

If one or more of the following conditions is present, consider risk as HIGH and it is necessary to proceed with task re-design.			
CRITICAL CONDITION: presence of lifting/carrying task lay-out and frequency conditions exceeding the maximum suggested			
VERTICAL LOCATION	The hand location at the beginning/end of the lift is higher than 175 cm or lower than 0 cm.	NO	YES
VERTICAL DISPLACEMENT	The vertical distance between the origin and the destination of the lifted object is more than 175 cm	NO	YES
HORIZONTAL DISTANCE	The horizontal distance between the body and load is greater than full arm reach	NO	YES
ASYMMETRY	Extreme body twisting without moving the feet	NO	YES
FREQUENCY	More than 15 lifts per min of SHORT DURATION (manual handling lasting no more than 60 min consecutively in the shift, followed by at least 60 minutes of break-light task)	NO	YES
	More than 12 lifts per min of MEDIUM DURATION (manual handling lasting no more than 120 min consecutively in the shift, followed by at least 30 minutes of break--light task)	NO	YES
	More than 8 lift per min of LONG DURATION (manual handling lasting more than 120 min consecutively in the shift)	NO	YES
CRITICAL CONDITION for lifting/carrying: presence of loads exceeding the following limits			
Males (18-45 years)	25 kg	NO	YES
Females (18-45 years)	20 kg	NO	YES
Males (<18 or >45 years)	20 kg	NO	YES
Females (<18 or >45 years)	15 kg	NO	YES
CRITICAL CONDITION FOR CARRYING: presence of cumulative carried mass greater than those indicated			
Carrying distance 20 m or more in 8 hours / Carrying distance per action 20 m or more	6000 kg in 8 hours	NO	YES
Carrying distance less than 20 m in 8 hours / Carrying distance per action less than 20 m	10000 kg in 8 hours	NO	YES
If at least one of the conditions have a "YES" response then a critical condition is present. If a critical condition is present then apply ISO 11228-1 for identifying urgent corrective actions.			

FIGURE 2.4   Lifting and carrying: Quick Assessment – critical conditions.

Figure 2.5 shows the preliminary conditions that must be examined in the case of whole-body *pushing and pulling*. It is important to note that if one or more of these preliminary conditions are inadequate, it cannot be established if the condition is fully acceptable or not, and steps must be taken to amend the inadequate conditions.

Moving on to acceptable conditions for *pushing and pulling*, Figure 2.6 shows a list of conditions that *must all be present simultaneously* in order to determine that the situation is acceptable (green).

In order to deal with the issue of quantifying the intensity of force, it is possible to make use of an indirect estimate through a "participatory" procedure that provides for the collection of data on the effort perceived by the worker(s) using the Borg CR-10 scale (Borg, 1998): this makes it possible to avoid performing a difficult instrumental measurement using a dynamometer.

Figure 2.7 shows the potential critical conditions for *pushing and pulling*; if even just one condition is present, the situation is defined as *critical*.

Working environment conditions		
Are floor surfaces slippery, not stable, uneven, have an upward or downward slope or are fissured, cracked or broken?	NO	YES
Are restricted or constrained movement paths present?	NO	YES
Is the temperature of the working area high	NO	YES
The characteristics of the object pushed or pulled		
Does the object (or trolley, transpallet, etc.) limit the vision of the operator or hinder the movement?	NO	YES
Is the object unstable?	NO	YES
Does the object (or trolley, transpallet, etc.) have hazardous features, sharp surfaces, projections etc. that can injure the operator?	NO	YES
Are the wheels or casters worn, broken or not properly maintained?	NO	YES
Are the wheels or casters unsuitable for the work conditions?	NO	YES
If the answers for all the conditions are "NO", then continue the quick assessment. If at least one of the answers is "YES", then apply ISO 11228-2. The consequent specific additional risks HAVE TO be carefully considered to MINIMIZE THESE RISKS.		

FIGURE 2.5 Pushing and pulling: preliminary aspects.

Hazard	Force magnitude		
	The force magnitude does not exceed approx. 30 N (or approximately 50 N for frequencies up to once per 5 min up to 50 m) for continuous (sustained) force exertion and approx. 100 N for peak (initial) force application. Alternatively, the perceived effort (obtained interviewing the workers using the CR-10 Borg scale) shows the presence, during the pushing-pulling task(s), of an up to SLIGHT force exertion (perceived effort) (score 2 or less in Borg CR-10 scale).	NO	YES
Hazard	**Task duration**		
	Does the task(s) with manual pushing and pulling last up to 8 hours a day?	NO	YES
Hazard	**Grasp height**		
	The push-or-pull force is applied to the object between hip and mid-chest level.	NO	YES
Hazard	**Posture**		
	The push-or-pull action is performed with an upright trunk (not twisted or bent).	NO	YES
Hazard	**Handling Area**		
	Hands are held inside shoulder width and in front of the body.	NO	YES
If all of the questions are answered "YES", then the examined task is in green area (ACCEPTABLE) and it is not necessary to continue the risk evaluation. If at least one of the questions is answered "NO", then evaluate the task(s) by ISO 11228-2.			

FIGURE 2.6 Lifting and carrying: Quick Assessment – critical conditions.

Here too, in order to quantify the intensity of force, it is possible to use the Borg CR-10 scale, thus making the Quick Assessment for the pushing and pulling entirely observational rather than instrumental.

With regard to repetitive tasks and ISO 11228-3, Figure 2.8 shows a list of conditions that must all be present simultaneously to evaluate a repetitive manual task as acceptable (green).

If a repetitive task is assessed as acceptable using the *Quick Assessment* procedure, this would be equivalent to classifying it as acceptable using the detailed methods indicated by the relevant standards.

If one or more of the following conditions is present, consider risk as HIGH, and it is necessary to proceed with task re-design.			
Hazard	**FORCE MAGNITUDE**		
	A) Peak initial force during push-or-pull (to overcome rest state (inertia) or to accelerate or to decelerate an object): The force is at least 360 N (males) or 240 N (females). B) Continuous (sustained) push-or-pull (to keep an object in motion): The force is at least 250 N (males) or 150 N (females) Alternatively, during the pushing-pulling task(s), the perceived effort using the CR-10 Borg scale (obtained by interviewing the workers), shows the presence of high peaks of force (perceived effort) (a score of 8 or more on the Borg CR-10 scale)?	NO	YES
Hazard	**POSTURE**		
	The push-or-pull action is performed with the trunk significantly bent or twisted.	NO	YES
Hazard	**FORCE EXERTION**		
	The push-or-pull action is performed in a jerky manner or in an uncontrolled way.	NO	YES
Hazard	**GRASP HANDLING AREA**		
	Hands are held either outside the shoulder width or not in front of the body.	NO	YES
Hazard	**GRASP HEIGHT**		
	Hands are held higher than 150 cm or lower than 60 cm.	NO	YES
Hazard	**FORCE DIRECTION**		
	The push-or-pull action is superimposed by relevant vertical force components ("partial lifting")	NO	YES
Hazard	**TASK DURATION**		
	Does the task(s) with manual pushing and pulling lasts more than 8 hours a day?	NO	YES
If one or more answers are "YES", then a critical condition is present. If a critical condition is present then apply ISO 11228-2 for identifying corrective actions.			

FIGURE 2.7   Pushing and pulling: Quick Assessment – critical conditions.

Conversely, Figure 2.9 lists situations which, even if they occur alone, will determine a critical condition.

To make a Quick Assessment of "*definitely critical*" conditions, reference has been made to the definitions and criteria included in the methods recommended by the standards (starting with the Occupational Repetitive Actions, OCRA, method), which indicate one or more highly risky elements. These might include very high-frequency actions using the upper limbs or repeated use of almost maximum force. If a repetitive manual handling condition is found to be critical, even in just one of the situations listed in Figure 2.9, the recommendation is to opt immediately for rapid and substantial remedial actions (risk reduction) without necessarily conducting a more in-depth analytical evaluation, which can,

Are either upper limbs working for less than 50% of the total time duration of repetitive task(s)?	NO	YES
Are both elbows held below the shoulder level for almost 90% of the total duration of the repetitive task(s)?	NO	YES
Is there a moderate force (perceived effort = max 3 or 4 on CR-10 Borg scale) exerted by the operator for no more than 1 hour during the duration of the repetitive task(s)?	NO	YES
Absence of force peaks (perceived effort = 5 or more on CR-10 Borg scale)	NO	YES
Presence of breaks (including the lunch break) that lasts at least 8 min every 2 hours?	NO	YES
Are the repetitive task(s) performed for less than 8 hours a day?	NO	YES

If all of the questions are answered "YES",
then the examined task is in Green area (ACCEPTABLE) and it is not necessary to continue the risk evaluation.
If at least one of the questions is answered "NO", then evaluate the task(s) by ISO 11228-3.

FIGURE 2.8 ISO/TR 12295: Quick Assessment for repetitive manual tasks: acceptability criteria (acceptable area).

If at least one of the following conditions is present (YES), the risk has to be considered as CRITICAL and it is necessary to proceed with URGENT task re-design.

Are technical actions of a single limb so fast that it cannot be counted by simple direct observation?	NO	YES
One or both arms are operating with the elbow at shoulder height for half or more than the total repetitive working time	NO	YES
A "pinch" grip (or all kinds of grasps using the fingers tips) is used for more than 80% of the repetitive working time.	NO	YES
Peak force applied (perceived effort = 5 or more in CR-10 Borg scale) for 10% or more of the total repetitive working time?	NO	YES
There is no more than one break (lunch break included) in a shift of 6-8 hours?	NO	YES
Total repetitive working time is exceeding 8 hours within a shift?	NO	YES

If at least one of the questions is answered "YES", then a critical condition is present.
If a critical condition is present, then apply ISO 11228-3 for identifying urgent corrective actions.

FIGURE 2.9 ISO/TR 12295: Quick Assessment for repetitive manual tasks: criteria for identifying critical conditions.

however, be carried out at a later stage to verify the potential effectiveness of the corrective measures put in place.

With regard to (static) working postures, the Quick Assessment proposed by ISO/TR 12295 only refers to the evaluation of a potentially acceptable condition (Figure 2.10), while it has not been possible to univocally define critical conditions due to the aforementioned lack of application experience in this area. As will be shown later when describing the ERGOCHECK tool, these difficulties have led to a diversified proposal in the *Quick Assessment* of working postures.

2.1.3 UPDATES OF ISO 11228-1

Standard ISO 11228-1 (ISO, 2003) is currently being revised.

In light of the Draft under discussion, the revision may involve, among other things, amendments or adjustments to the parts relating to the Quick Assessment procedures for lifting and carrying, which are presented here as contained in ISO/TR 12295 of 2014.

Head and trunk evaluation		
Are both the trunk posture AND the neck posture symmetrical?	NO	YES
Is the trunk flexion to the front less than 20° OR in case of backward inclination, is the trunk fully supported?	NO	YES
Is there trunk flexion between 20° and 60°, AND is the trunk fully supported?	NO	YES
Is neck extension absent OR in case of neck flexion, is it less than 25°?	NO	YES
Is backward head inclination fully supported OR, in case of head inclination to the front, is it less than 25°?	NO	YES
If sitting, is a convex spinal curvature absent?	NO	YES
Upper limb evaluation (evaluate the more loaded limb)		
Right/Left		
Are awkward upper arm postures absent?	NO	YES
Are the shoulders not raised?	NO	YES
Without full arm support, is the upper arm elevation less than 20°?	NO	YES
With full arm support, is there upper arm elevation up to 60°?	NO	YES
Are extreme elbow flexion/extension AND extreme forearm rotation absent?	NO	YES
Is extreme wrist deviation absent?	NO	YES
Lower limb evaluation (evaluate the more loaded limb)		
Right/Left		
Is extreme knee flexion absent?	NO	YES
Is the knee not flexed in standing postures?	NO	YES
Is there a neutral ankle position?	NO	YES
Is kneeling or crouching absent?	NO	YES
When sitting, is the knee angle between 90° and 135°?	NO	YES
If all of the questions are answered "YES", then the examined task is in Green area (ACCEPTABLE), and is not necessary to continue the risk evaluation. If at least one of the questions is answered "NO", then evaluate the task(s) by ISO 11226.		

FIGURE 2.10   ISO/TR 12295: Quick Assessment for static postures: acceptability criteria (acceptable area).

Since nothing has so far been finalized and it is not known when the revised standard will be released, reference is made here to a few major changes (in relation to the Quick Assessment of Lifting and Carrying) that could be included in the new version of the standard, in which case the data collection worksheets and software presented here would need amending.

- The definition of "young" would not be below 18 years, but below 20 years; consequently, the reference weights of 20 kg for young males and 15 kg for young females (indicated as critical in the Quick Assessment form) are valid up to 20 years of age.
- Also in the Quick Assessment worksheet for critical conditions, when defining the critical conditions relating to lifting frequency and with reference to long durations (more than two continuous hours), critical frequency should increase from "more than 8 lifts per minute" to "more than 10 lifts per minute". This would ensure greater consistency with the frequency/duration multipliers provided by the same ISO 11228-1 standard (ISO, 2003), which would be confirmed.
- A more significant change might concern the Quick Assessment (for both acceptable and critical conditions) for carrying.

It is worth noting that in the assessment of carrying tasks, the new standard under discussion, confirming that it refers to the concept of a cumulative mass carried over a period of time, should provide new criteria for calculating the relevant limits in relation to minutes, individual hours (from 1 to 6 hours) and the whole shift (6–8 hours). The new criteria largely derive from a French standard on the same subject, adjusted for the limited amount of literature on the subject.

The limits provided by the standard (e.g., cumulative mass carried = 6,000 kg for 6–8 hours, 2,500 kg for 1 hour, 75 kg for 1 minute) are valid for a reference condition of flat ground and weight carried for a distance of up to 2 m, with suitable grip height, good environmental conditions and comfortable grip. If the actual conditions differ from those indicated, appropriate multipliers (or reduction factors) must be used depending on the degree of deviation from the reference condition. For example, if the scenario under examination involves carrying a load over a distance (average or modal) of between 5 and 10 m, the limits indicated for the reference scenario (2 m) must all be reduced by a factor of 0.6.

A Quick Assessment worksheet for carrying has been proposed with respect to these general criteria.

The worksheet includes the criteria shown in Table 2.1 for acceptable conditions.

TABLE 2.1
Carrying: Quick Assessment of Acceptable Conditions in the Draft for Revision of ISO 11228-1

	Calculate CUMULATIVE MASS (total kg carried for different durations and over different distances) Is the CUMULATIVE MASS LESS THAN or EQUAL to the RECOMMENDED CUMULATIVE MASS considering distance (more or less than 5 m) and distance (1 minute, 1 hour, 4 hours, 8 hours)?			
Duration	**Distance from 1 to ≤5 m per carrying task**	**Distance from >5 to 10 m per carrying task**		
6–8 hours	4.8 kg	3.6 kg	NO	YES
4 hours	4.0 kg	3.0 kg	NO	YES
1 hour	2.0 kg	1.5 kg	NO	YES
1 minute	60 kg	45 kg	NO	YES
	ACCEPTABLE CONDITIONS: Carrying a load with both hands over a distance of less than 10 m, picking up and putting down an object at a height of between 0.75 and 1.10 m, in a complete cycle that includes returning to the starting point over the same distance (empty-handed). The carrying task is performed in a comfortable indoor setting, on a hard, smooth and non-slippery floor; there are no obstacles in the way and the work space does not restrict posture or movement. There is no pre-set pace and no significantly awkward postures during carrying.		NO	YES
	If all the replies to these questions are "YES"			
	then the CARRYING TASK is ACCEPTABLE and no further assessment is required. If at least one reply to these questions is "NO" then the assessment must be continued.			

The criteria for critical conditions are shown in Table 2.2.

TABLE 2.2

Carrying: Quick Assessment of Critical Conditions in the Draft for Revision of ISO 11228-1

CRITICAL CONDITIONS FOR MANUAL CARRYING: Presence of cumulative loads weighing over the recommended level for conditions defined as acceptable in the previous table (Table 2.1)			
Carrying distance from 1 to 5 m for 6–8 hours?	6.0 tons in 6–8 hours	NO	YES
Carrying distance from 5 to 10 m for 6–8 hours?	3.6 tons in 6–8 hours	NO	YES
Carrying distance from 10 to 20 m for 6–8 hours?	1.2 tons in 6–8 hours	NO	YES
Carrying distance more than 20 m	Carrying distance usually over 20 m	NO	YES
If the reply to at least one of the above conditions is "YES" then the result is a CRITICAL CARRYING CONDITION If the carrying condition is CRITICAL, urgent corrective actions are necessary (see Annex A to the standard).			

2.2 REFERENCE SOURCES FOR THE PRELIMINARY STUDY OF BIOLOGICAL RISK

Ugo Caselli et al.
INAIL

Biological risk is defined as when workers, as part of their duties, may come into contact with biological agents, i.e., micro-organisms such as viruses, bacteria, fungi and parasites, which can affect the health of the workers themselves, or determine the onset of specific diseases. Micro-organisms, which vary considerably from the morphological, metabolic and pathological point of view, can be found in virtually all environments and in many different matrices and substrates, displaying a remarkable ability to adapt, colonize and spread. The management of biological risk therefore raises numerous critical issues, also in light of the vast range of modern production cycles and the characteristics of individual workers, who differ in age, gender, lifestyles and health conditions (INAIL, 2011; Sarto et al., 2018).

2.2.1 GENERAL INFORMATION REGARDING BIOLOGICAL AGENTS

2.2.1.1 Bacteria

Bacteria, which first appeared 3.5–3.7 billion years ago, were the first life forms on our planet and, in fact, are the least complex of all living cells, still consisting of an extremely large group of micro-organisms with different shapes, sizes and metabolisms. Bacteria are formed by a single cell and are able to live autonomously. They measure only a few microns in diameter and their shape depends on the species: they may be spherical (cocci), rod-shaped (bacilli) or curved (spirilla). Bacteria may exist as individual cells, or in clusters, sometimes with a characteristic shape, as in the case of streptococci, which are round bacteria that form chains, or staphylococci, which are also round, but are clustered randomly in groups. Bacterial cells usually have a rigid outer layer called the cell wall, below which lies the cytoplasmic membrane that encloses the cytoplasm (cytosol), which contains certain specific organelles, as well as the cell's DNA. The cytoplasm is where all the cell's vital functions are concentrated. There may be appendages attached to the surface of bacteria, known as flagella, fimbriae or pili. Flagella are strand-like organisms that enable the bacterial cell to move. Their number and arrangement depend on the species. They are larger in size than pili, which enable bacteria to conjugate (or reproduce). DNA containing genetic information takes the shape of a round molecule in the cytoplasm, anchored to the cytoplasmatic membrane. Some bacterial species produce spores, enabling them to survive in temporarily unfavorable conditions; once conditions are again favorable, the spore develops into a normal cell. Metabolically, bacteria are highly flexible: they can acquire energy through various processes, such as cellular respiration, photosynthesis and the fermentation of organic compounds. Thanks to their ability to synthesize most of the components they need, starting from simple compounds such as water, carbon dioxide, nitrogen, phosphorus, etc., bacteria have colonized every environment, even adapting to extreme conditions and accounting for almost 50% of the biomass of earth's living organisms. The versatility of bacteria is further proven by their metabolism's ability to utilize oxygen (aerobes), although many species can live without oxygen (anaerobes) or in low-oxygen environments. Bacteria can be harmful to human health, with severity depending on factors such as the species and strain, the health status of the host, the presence of matrices or substrates that enable them to spread, and so on. Over the century, mankind has been tormented by diseases such as the plague, cholera and tuberculosis, which have caused many thousands if not millions of deaths due to certain species of bacteria. Some, like the plague and cholera, have been quelled, while others, like tuberculosis, have made subtle but more dangerous reappearances, through the selection of antibiotic-resistant bacterial strains.

2.2.1.2 Viruses

Viruses do not have a cellular architecture as they are comprised only of nucleic acid, either DNA or RNA, featuring a variety of different structures (single-stranded or double-stranded, linear or circular) and proteins that coat the genetic material, called capsids. They are generally much smaller than bacteria, their dimensions being in the order of nanometers, and they have a helical or icosahedral structure. Viruses have a protein coating that both protects the nucleic acid from degradation due to the extracellular environment and enables the virus to adhere to specific receptors on the cytoplasmic membrane of the host cell. Viruses have no metabolic functions and are unable to reproduce autonomously; being obligatory intracellular parasites, they grow and can only reproduce in the cells of specific hosts, which may be animals, plants, fungi, etc. Viral replication begins with attachment or adsorption between the virus and the host cell membrane. The virus particle then enters the cell and releases nucleic acid, which begins to express itself. This triggers intense metabolic activity in the cell to enable the expression of the viral genome, its replication and the production of structural proteins that then build new viruses. Ultimately, viral particles are released by the host cell when the cell ruptures or by budding at the outer cytoplasmic membrane. Viral offspring then infect new host cells. Many viruses are harmful to humans, and some are extremely widespread, such as those that cause childhood exanthematous diseases (such as measles, rubella, etc.), influenza and parainfluenza viruses and hepatitis viruses (A, B, C, etc.); others are less known and are localized in specific geographical areas (e.g., Ebola). The diseases that they cause in humans present very different symptoms and may vary in severity from colds and influenza to life-threatening conditions like hepatitis, Acquired Immune Deficiency Syndrome (AIDS), etc.

2.2.1.3   Fungi

Fungi are multicellular heterotrophic organisms that feed by absorption. Fungi are eukaryotes and are protected externally by a cell wall composed of chitin. The eukaryotic cell has a cytoplasmic membrane that encloses the cytoplasm; immersed in the cytoplasm are structures known as organelles, as well as the nucleus. The cytoplasmic membrane is comprised of a double layer of phospholipids and is semipermeable, allowing the direct passage of small molecules, such as sugars and salts, while larger molecules are transported by active transport systems. The cytoplasm, unlike in the prokaryotic cell, contains numerous organelles, each with its own specific structure and function, through which metabolic functions are compartmentalized; each function is performed most efficiently in a specific organelle. The genetic material of the eukaryotic cell is mainly contained in the nucleus, where DNA duplication and transcription and RNA maturation take place. Fungi, although multicellular, do not have differentiated tissues; they have a heterotrophic diet and feed on organic substances processed by other organisms. Fungi are made up of unicellular or multicellular thread-like filaments that may be uninucleate or polynucleate, with an elongated cylindrical shape, called hyphae, which, placed one on top of the other, form the mycelium, the vegetative body of the fungus. Depending on their nutritional needs, fungi are divided into saprophytes, parasites and symbionts or mutualistic. Saprophytes degrade non-living substances of animal or plant origin into less complex compounds, parasites feed on living organisms, while symbionts are a form of controlled parasitism in which a fungus benefits from the host and the host also benefits from the fungus, creating a mutualistic type of relationship. Many species of fungi cause human diseases, such as candida, which give rise to opportunistic infections in immunocompromised patients, and the genus Aspergillus, which causes disease by producing mycotoxins, inducing allergic responses and developing localized or systemic infections.

2.2.1.4   Parasites

The term **parasite** refers not to a specific group from the systematic point of view, but rather to a set of living organisms that complete some or all of their life cycle in different animal species and belong to morphologically and metabolically diverse groups. All parasites, however, can live at the expense of other species, generally causing harm in infected individuals. Some parasites invade specific tissues or organs, some produce toxins that are harmful to the host, while others rob nutrients from the host organism, thus causing weakness and depression. The parasite does not only feed off its host but uses the host as its own ecological niche. From the morphological standpoint, parasites can be classified as unicellular or multicellular organisms, while on the basis of their life cycle, it is possible to identify facultative parasites, which can live independently from the host, and obligate parasites, which depend entirely on the host. The host may be permanent, when the parasite lives its entire life within or on the host, or temporary, when the parasite lives free of its host during part of its life cycle. Ectoparasites infest the skin of the host (e.g. lice, fleas, mites, ticks, etc.). Endoparasites live in the body of the host (e.g. protozoa, worms, etc.). Malaria, toxoplasmosis, hookworm and tapeworm are just some of the diseases caused by endoparasites in humans. Malaria, undoubtedly the most widespread of all parasites and the second most lethal disease in the world, is caused by protozoa of the genus Plasmodium: infected individuals are their reservoir and the mosquitoes of the genus Anopheles are their vector. Parasites have a very complicated life cycle that involves mosquitoes and human hosts, particularly their circulatory and digestive system.

2.2.2   EUROPEAN AND ITALIAN LEGISLATION CONCERNING EXPOSURE TO BIOLOGICAL AGENTS

In Europe, European Directive 2000/54/EC still applies and has been transposed into the legislation of various EU member countries: Italy transposed the directive into Legislative Decree no. 81 in 2008. The EU Directive is a later version of European Directive 1990/679/EEC, which was the first European regulation to address the issue of biological risk in the workplace.

European Directive 2000/54/EC specifies that biological risk, as well as other health and safety risks, must be assessed in the workplace in order to determine the most suitable management and control methods, based on the latest scientific evidence. The Directive indicates the scope, definitions and classification of biological agents, the obligations of the employer, health and safety monitoring and, lastly, the penalties for non-compliance.

The Directive applies to all jobs where there is a risk of exposure to biological agents, in particular to any job that involves the deliberate use, i.e., the intentional introduction into the production cycle, of biological agents that are used, handled, transformed or exploited for their intrinsic biological properties. It also applies to any activity where there may be potential or accidental exposure to micro-organisms randomly present in the working environment, which could harm the worker's health.

"Biological agent" refers to any micro-organism, including if it is genetically modified, or cell culture, or human endoparasite that can cause infections, allergies or toxicity.

"Micro-organisms" are defined as any microbiological entity, both cellular and non-cellular, capable of replication or of transferring genetic material, while "cell culture" is the result of the in-vitro growth of cells deriving from multicellular organisms.

Biological agents can cause infection, i.e., a pathological reaction of the host, following the entry, development and multiplication of micro-organisms; they may lead to intoxication through the ingestion of substances that are toxic in nature or dosage, in the form of acute or chronic states, and may cause allergies, which are excessive reactions driven by particular antibodies against substances that are usually harmless and are biologically derived.

Biological agents are classified into four groups on the basis of their degree of hazard for the health of the human host and, in particular, of workers: infectivity, pathogenicity, transmissibility and neutralizability. This classification enables risk containment levels to be determined and measures to be adopted based on measuring the hazard level of the group of micro-organisms involved.

Infectivity is the ability of a micro-organism to enter and multiply in a susceptible host; it is inversely proportional to the number of micro-organisms required to establish infection in a given host and depends on different variables, such as environmental conditions, transmission pathways, the health status of the host and, last but not least, the species and strain to which the micro-organism belongs.

The infectivity threshold or minimum infectious dose, i.e., the minimum amount of biological agent capable of experimentally inducing a disease, which is difficult to determine, is known for a small number of agents. For the purposes of risk assessment, it is conservatively assumed that the minimum infectious dose is 1 for all biological agents.

Pathogenicity is the ability of a micro-organism to induce a disease process; it is genetically determined and is measured by the degree of virulence.

Transmissibility indicates the micro-organism's ability to spread within the human population by transmission from infected to healthy susceptible individuals. Transmission may occur by:

- Direct contact between subjects, one of whom is affected by the disease and the other is healthy, with the physical transfer of the micro-organism from one to another (e.g. diseases transmitted from mother to fetus or sexually transmitted infections).
- Indirect contact, when a vector or carrier acts as an intermediary host is between the two subjects. Vectors include air, water, but also objects, equipment and devices in common use, if contaminated.
- By means of vectors that are living creatures that carry micro-organisms and disseminate them into the external environment, through inoculation in the host; example include certain species of ticks and mosquitoes.

Neutralizability depends on whether or not effective prophylactic measures to prevent the disease, such as vaccines or treatments, are available.

Biological agents are classified according to European Directive 2000/54/EC into four groups:

- Group 1 includes organisms with a low likelihood of causing disease in humans.
- Group 2 includes agents that may cause disease in humans and be a risk to workers, but are unlikely to spread to communities; effective prophylactic and therapeutic measures are generally available.

- Group 3 includes agents that can cause serious diseases in humans and pose a serious risk to workers; the agent can spread to communities, but effective prophylactic and therapeutic measures are usually available.
- Group 4 includes agents that can cause serious diseases in humans and pose a serious risk to workers; there is a high risk of spreading to communities; in this case, effective prophylactic or therapeutic measures are not available.

Figure 2.11 shows some examples of micro-organisms belonging to groups 2, 3 and 4 (Annex 3 of European Directive 2000/54/EC).

Figure 2.11 shows that groups 2 and 3 include many species of bacteria, viruses, fungi and parasites, while group 4 is comprised exclusively of viruses. This classification is based on the effects of biological agents on healthy workers, but does not take into account many worker-specific variables, such as age, gender, lifestyle, health status, etc.

Employers are required to assess exposure to biological agents based on a substantial amount of information comprised principally of:

- Tasks entailing exposure to biological agents;
- Number of workers considered to be exposed;
- Preventative and protective measures implemented;
- Emergency procedures in place.

Moreover, the employer is obliged to know which biological agents workers are exposed to, as well as to classify the agents and the diseases or disorders they may cause, potential allergic and toxic effects, and any diseases or disorders reported by workers that might be related to their job.

Regarding the technical, organizational and procedural measures to be adopted in the event that the assessment reveals risks for workers, it is essential to avoid the use of harmful biological agents, design work processes so as to achieve that aim,

BIOLOGICAL AGENT				
Group	Bacteria	Virus	Fungi	Parasites
2	Bordetella pertussis; Borrelia spp.; Campylobacter spp.; Clostridium botulinum; Clostridium tetani; Corynebacterium spp.; Enterobacter spp.; Klebsiella spp.; Legionella pneumophila; Neisseria meningitides; Rickettsia spp.; Staphylococcus aureus; Streptococcus pyogenes; Vibrio cholerae.	Adenoviridae; Cytomegalovirus; Epstein-Barr virus; Human herpesvirus 3; Herpes simplex virus 1 and 2; Influenza A, B and C virus; Measles morbillivirus; Parotitis virus; Human parainfluenza viruses; Poliovirus; Human rotavirus.	Aspergillus fumigatus; Candida albicans; Sporothrix schenckii; Trichophyton spp.	Ancylostoma duodenale; Cryptosporidium spp.; Giardia lamblia; Taenia saginata; Toxoplasma gondii.
3	Bacillus anthracis; Brucella melitensis; Mycobacterium tuberculosis; Salmonella typhi; Yersinia pestis.	HBV; HCV; Dengue virus; Yellow fever virus; Nile Valley virus; AIDS; Rabies virus.	Coccidioides immitis; Histoplasma capsulatum.	Echinococcus granulosus; Leishmania brasiliensis; Plasmodium falciparum; Taenia solium
4	-	Ebola virus; Marburg virus.	-	-

FIGURE 2.11 A selection of micro-organisms belonging to groups 2, 3 and 4, identified in Annex III to Directive 2000/54/CE.

adopt collective/individual protective measures and health and hygiene measures, put in place procedures for obtaining, handling and processing samples of human and animal origin, define emergency procedures for dealing with accidents, manage waste safely, and take any other necessary precautions.

As regards health and hygiene, workers must have adequate washing facilities at their disposal, including showers and, if necessary, eye washes and antiseptic hand rubs, along with protective clothing and other suitable gear, which should be stored separately from their everyday clothing; personal protective equipment must be provided as needed.

Specific measures must be adopted for healthcare services and laboratories, animal enclosures and industrial processes, and particular attention must be paid to biological agents potentially released by patients or animals or contained in samples and residues, and to the risks that such agents may represent for certain tasks. Workers must receive on-going education and training regarding exposure to biological risk, especially the precautions to be taken to avoid exposure, good hygiene practices, the purpose and proper use of protective gear and equipment, how to prevent workplace accidents and what to do to minimize the consequences.

Following exposure to biological agents, adequate health surveillance must be put in place before the next exposure, and repeated at regular intervals.

2.2.3   EUROPEAN LEGISLATION CONCERNING THE PREVENTION OF NEEDLE-STICK INJURIES AND CUTS IN THE HOSPITAL AND HEALTHCARE SECTOR

European Directive 2010/32/EU concerns the prevention of needle-stick injuries and cuts in the hospital and healthcare sector; the Directive was assimilated into Italian law with Legislative Decree 81/08.

"Sharp" is the term used to describe objects or instruments necessary for the exercise of specific healthcare activities, which are able to cut, prick or infect the user. The employer must therefore consider whether workers may be injured when using these instruments. In addition, the employer must determine the necessary technical, organizational and procedural measures to ensure safe working conditions, the level of professional qualifications, work-related psychosocial factors and the influence of the working environment. This emphasizes the fact that the risk of pricks and cuts may also depend on organizational factors (e.g. shifts) or psychosocial factors (e.g. work-related stress). Workers must suitably trained. Specific preventative measures to be taken include doing away with the unnecessary use of sharp instruments or tools, establishing and implementing safe utilization and disposal procedures for medical sharps (which cannot be eliminated from the work cycle) and waste contaminated with high-risk blood or biological materials, and ensuring the installation of properly marked and technically safe containers for handling and disposing of medical sharps and disposable needles as close as possible to the areas where sharps or sharp objects are used or stored.

2.2.4   BIOLOGICAL AGENTS IN MANUFACTURING SECTORS

Workers may be exposed to biological agents used deliberately in specific production cycles; such agents have intrinsic characteristics that make them an integral part of the process.

Similarly, workers may be exposed to biological agents found occasionally or accidentally in the workplace, also due to various factors such as, for example, the presence of raw materials, the type of production cycle, hygiene in the working environment, etc.

The variety and diversity of sectors and processes existing today pose many challenges for effective risk management with regard to biological agents in the primary, secondary and tertiary sectors. Figure 2.12 shows examples of biological agents found in different production sectors, along with an indication of the pathologies that they cause.

2.2.5 ASSESSMENT OF THE RISK OF EXPOSURE TO BIOLOGICAL AGENTS

European Directive 2000/54/EC stresses the need to implement a number of steps, starting from a proper risk assessment, in order to eliminate/reduce risk by adopting suitable and appropriate prevention and protection measures, and also by providing training and health surveillance programs for workers.

In particular, it emphasizes that the **risk assessment phase** must cover tasks/activities that involve the deliberate and non-deliberate use of biological agents and take into account all the information that are essential for a proper assessment, such as the type of biological agents deliberately used and/or potentially present in the task or job, the diseases that they may cause, the tasks or steps in the work process that involve exposure to biological agents, the number of workers exposed and their health status, etc. It is therefore obvious that a large amount of information needs to be recorded in order to better address the risk assessment phase, although it is arguably very difficult to combine the information and ultimately reach preliminary conclusions that are sufficiently representative of the level of risk involved. Unlike other types of risk, there are currently no clearly defined limits for exposure to biological agents, precisely because the subject is so difficult to integrate the many factors that contribute to the spread of a pathogen and the development of an infection. This explains why the assessment of biological risk is anything but simple and why there is as yet no standard procedure for formulating a precise estimate of this risk.

A conceptually similar approach to the one set out in European Directive 2000/54/EC has been adopted by the Center of Disease Control and Prevention in Atlanta (USA) (CDC, 2018).

The European Agency for Safety & Health at Work (EU-OSHA, 2010) states that risk assessments should be carried out in five successive steps:

- Step 1: identify the hazards and subsequently the risk, by searching the workplace for potential sources of hazard, and identify potentially exposed workers.
- Step 2: assess and define priorities by estimating risks in terms of their severity and likelihood to cause harm.
- Step 3: define appropriate preventative measures for eliminating or controlling risk.
- Step 4: plan and put preventative and protective measures in place based on priorities.
- Step 5: monitor and re-examine.

BIOLOGICAL AGENTS (PATHOLOGY) BY OCCUPATIONAL SECTOR

AGRICULTURE, FORESTRY	ANIMAL HUSBANDRY	LIVESTOCK SLAUGHTER AND MEAT PROCESSING	PROCESSING AND DISPOSAL OF SOLID AND LIQUID WASTE
Borrelia burgdorferi (Lyme disease); Brucella spp. (brucellosis); Clostridium tetani (tetanus); Coxiella burnetii (Q fever); Escherichia coli (intestinal infections); Francisella tularensis (tularaemia); Rickettsia spp. (rickettsiosis); Salmonella spp. (salmonellosis); Shigella spp. (intestinal infections); Arbovirus (arbovirosis); Enterovirus (gastrointestinal tract infections); Phlebovirus (encephalitis, haemorrhagic fever); Alternaria alternata (allergies); Aspergillus spp. (respiratory tract infections); Sporotrix scheckii (sporotrichosis); Ancylostoma duodenalis (hookworms); Mites (allergic dermatitis).	Bacillus anthracis (anthrax); Borrelia burgdorferi (Lyme disease); Brucella spp. (brucellosis); Campylobacter spp. (campylobacteriosis); Coxiella burnetii (Q fever); Clostridium tetani (tetanus); Helycobacter spp. (gastric infection); Francisella tularensis (tularaemia); Leptospira interrogans (leptospirosis); Listeria monocytogenens (listeriosis); Mycobacterium spp. (tuberculosis); Salmonella spp. (salmonellosis); Rickettsia conorii (rickettsiosis); Yersinia spp. (plague); Streptococcus suis (various infections); Orthomyxovirus (influenza); Papovavirus (neoplastic proliferations); Poxvirus (contagious mollusc); Rhabdovirus (rabies); Trichophyton spp. (dermatomycosis); Echinococcus spp. (Echinococcosis)	Bacillus anthracis (anthrax); Brucella spp. (brucellosis); Campylobacter spp. (campylobacteriosis); Coxiella burnetii (Q fever); Clostridium tetani (tetanus); Helycobacter spp. (gastric infection); Leptospira interrogans (leptospirosis); Listeria monocytogenans (listeriosis); Mycobacterium spp. (tuberculosis); Salmonella spp. (salmonellosis); Rickettsia conorii (rickettsiosis); HAV (hepatitis A); Orthomyxovirus (influenza); Papillomavirus (warts); Poxvirus (molluscum contagiosum); Penicillium spp. (mycosis); Echinococcus spp. (echinococcosis); Toxoplasma gondii (toxoplasmosis); Ascaris lumbricoides (ascaridiasi); Mites (allergic dermatitis).	Clostridium tetanes (tetanus); Escherichia coli (intestinal infections); Leptospira interrogans (leptospirosis); Salmonella spp. (salmonellosis); Enterobacter spp. (urinary tract infections); HAV (hepatitis A); Enterovirus (GI infections); Rotavirus (gastroenteritis); Cytomegalovirus (various infections); Alternaria alternata (allergies); Aspergillus spp. (respiratory tract infections); Penicillium spp. (mycosis); Ascaris spp. (ascariasis); Giardia intestinalis (giardiasis or beaver fever).

HOSPITALS, NURSING HOMES AND LABORATORIES	BUILDING CONSTRUCTION	CLEANING AND DISINFECTION COMPANIES	PUBLIC HEALTH AND WELFARE, DESK JOBS
Bordetella pertussis (pertussis or whooping cough); Brucella spp. (brucellosis); Legionella pneumophyla (legionellosis); Mycobacterium spp. (tuberculosis); Neisseria meningitidis (meningitis); Pseudomonas aeruginosa (various infections); Salmonella spp. (salmonellosis); Staphylococcus aureus (various infections); Streptococcus pyogenes (various infections); HIV (AIDS); HBV (hepatitis B); HCV (hepatitis C); Herpesvirus (various infections); Toxoplasma gondii (toxoplasmosis); Mites (allergic dermatitis).	Borrelia burgdoleri (Lyme disease); Clostridium tetans (tetanus); Leptospira interrogans (leptospirosis); Legionella pneumophyla (legionellosis); Salmonella spp. (salmonellosis); Aspergillus spp. (respiratory tract infections); Penicillium spp. (mycosis); Alternaria alternata (allergies); HBV (hepatitis B); HCV (hepatitis C); Enterovirus (GI infections); Ascaris spp. (ascariasis); Ancylostoma duodenale (ankylostomiasis).	Legionella pneumophyla (legionellosis); Staphylococcus spp. (various infections); Streptococcus spp. (various infections); HBV (hepatitis B); HCV (hepatitis C); HIV (AIDS); Papillomavirus (warts); Enterovirus (GI infections); Trichophyton spp. (dermatomycosis); Mites (allergic dermatitis).	Legionella pneumophyla (legionellosis); Staphylococcus spp. (various infections); Rhinovirus (colds); Influenza viruses (flu); Alternaria alternata (allergies); Aspergillus spp. (respiratory tract infections); Penicillium spp. (mycosis); Mites (allergic dermatitis).

FIGURE 2.12   Examples of biological agents not used deliberately in various working sectors.

The evaluation should take into account the latest scientific evidence, best practices and techniques. Based on the results, the employer should establish the necessary levels of containment, a schedule, a list of measures to be implemented, including training and information, and control and health monitoring procedures. EU-OSHA offers a checklist for this purpose, specifying that it is a practical, non-exhaustive method for identifying hazards and prevention measures, and forms at least a preliminary part of the biological risk assessment.

Sarto et al. (2018) developed a methodology based on an algorithm for assessing biological risk which, unlike other methods, quantifies all the factors affecting biological risk, also based on numerous indications found in the technical literature, in order to reach a final estimate of the risk level for workers.

2.2.6 Measures for Preventing Exposure to Biological Agents

Once potential exposure to biological agents has been assessed by analyzing the various critical factors mentioned above, the most appropriate risk prevention measures must be implemented. General measures include eliminating the source of risk represented by the biological pathogen, if feasible. If the biological agent is deliberately used in the production cycle, it should be replaced by another non-pathogenic agent. If the biological agent is potentially present in the workplace, it is essential to eliminate whatever factors encourage its existence. If the biological agent cannot be eliminated, it must be confined to reduce the number of potentially exposed workers. The implementation of suitable hygiene measures in the workplace, however, can significantly minimize risk. Workers must be provided with information and training, primarily to ensure that the most suitable operating procedures and behaviors are adopted. Certain working environments, especially hospitals, also require the implementation of numerous preventative measures that may differ substantially depending on the characteristics of the workplace, but which are all designed to reduce risk.

Disinfection and sterilization procedures are the mainstays of risk prevention in the workplace: disinfection aims to eliminate or drastically reduce the presence of harmful micro-organisms, while sterilization seeks to destroy all living organisms in a given substrate or environment. These procedures can be carried out by means of physical methods, such as ultraviolet radiation, heat, steam, etc., and/or the use of chemicals such as compounds that may include chlorine, bromine, hydrogen peroxide, alcohols, aldehydes, ethylene oxide, etc. Disinfection and/or sterilization can be used on substrates, objects and whole rooms. Effective forms of prevention can also be implemented on people and workers through prophylactic immunization, which determines specific resistance to a certain pathogen. Prophylactic immunization is defined as active when vaccines are administered and passive when immune sera and immunoglobulins are used. Depending on the disease, vaccines may be an effective solution, while in other cases they need to be used in conjunction with other preventative measures.

2.2.7   COLLECTIVE AND INDIVIDUAL PROTECTION MEASURES AGAINST BIOLOGICAL AGENTS

After implementing every possible preventive measure (i.e., doing away with or reducing hazards, containing the number of exposed workers, etc.), if a residual risk remains, the employer must put in place systems aimed at protecting workers against the risks to which they are exposed. Protective equipment may be divided into collective (CPE) and personal (PPE); the legislator places collective protection at a higher priority than personal protective measures.

Generally speaking, collective protective equipment (CPE) is directed against the source of emission of the pollutant, and acts by eliminating or reducing the contamination of the working environment and consequently the risk of contact between the pollutant and the worker. For protection against exposure to biological agents, it is possible to capture the air flow at the point of emission, along with biological particles and polluting aerosols produced during the work activity (i.e., with localized systems or measures), and then remove the pollutants with high efficiency particulate air (HEPA) filters. It is also possible to dilute the pollutant or shift the polluted air mass by introducing clean air into the working environment. Other systems include biological safety hoods and insulators.

In the event that prevention and collective protection systems are unable to provide effective protection of the worker's health, PPE plays a fundamental role. PPE is defined as "any equipment intended to be worn for the purpose of protecting the worker against one or more risks likely to threaten his or her safety or health at work, as well as any ancillary equipment intended for that purpose". PPE must be correctly used and maintained, as specified by the product technical standards.

PPEs have been divided at the European level into three risk categories (Regulation EU 2016/425):

- Category I, designed to protect users against minimal risks (superficial injuries, contact with mildly aggressive chemicals, etc.);
- Category II, PPE other than those included in groups I and III;
- Category III, designed to protect users against risks that may cause very serious consequences such as irreversible damage to health injury or death (e.g., protection of the respiratory tract against hazardous biological agents); training is compulsory.

Since contact with biological agents can occur through the skin, mucous membranes and airways, accidental ingestion or parenterally via scratches and insect bites, it is necessary to use the most suitable specific PPEs for preventing the various modes of infection.

It is possible to protect the face and airways, especially from bioaerosols, using face shields, goggles, filtering face-pieces and filter respirators.

To protect the hands, gloves made out of different materials can be used, such as latex, vinyl, nitrile, and of different thicknesses, to protect the user from pathogens that are transmissible by contact.

Disposable bodysuits or gowns protect the body, while safety footwear, including purpose-made shoes, overshoes and boots are useful for protecting the lower limbs.

2.3 REFERENCE SOURCES FOR THE STUDY OF WORK-RELATED STRESS: STANDARDS AND BEST PRACTICES FOR THE PRELIMINARY ASSESSMENT, MANAGEMENT AND PREVENTION OF RISK

Paolo Campanini
Ergonomics of Posture and Movements International Ergonomics School (EPM-IES)

Alberto Baratti
Territorial and hospital occupational medicine services at ASL CN 1 Ergonomics of Posture and Movements International Ergonomics School (EPM-IES)

2.3.1 FROM THE EUROPEAN FRAMEWORK AGREEMENT OF 2004 TO ITALY'S LEGISLATIVE DECREE 81/08

Under the heading "Purpose of risk assessment", Article 28.1 of Legislative Decree 81/08, recites as follows:

> The assessment referred to in Article 17.1a must cover all risks to the health and safety of workers, including groups of workers exposed to particular risks, where risks refer also to work-related stress under the meaning of the **European Framework Agreement of 8 October 2004**.

Therefore, with reference to this particular risk factor, Italian legislators have enacted a law that requires employers to carry out risk assessments pursuant to the contents of the European Framework Agreement (ETUC et al., 2004), but does not require them to adopt a particular assessment methodology. It is worth noting that Italian lawmakers have laid down such clear-cut and explicit instructions as these in relation to only a very small number of other risk factors (pertaining to, for example, working mothers, and physical and ergonomic risk).

The European Framework Agreement ("Agreement") establishes a number of basic standards for risk assessment, and thus serves as a sort of regulatory-methodological point of reference for risk assessment (as distinct from a scientific one, since it is merely a framework document) that explicitly gives employers ample leeway to choose their own assessment methods and tools as long as they are compliant with the model postulated in the Agreement:

> The aim of the present Agreement is to provide employers and workers with a framework to identify and prevent or manage problems of work-related stress.

The following basic tenets of the European Agreement of 2004 were transposed into Italian law through Legislative Decree 81/08:

- Stress can affect any workplace and any worker... therefore the risk assessment must involve all companies, irrespective of their size or field of activity.
- It is essential to allow for the different characteristics of workers.

- Not all workplaces and not all workers are affected by stress, and not all manifestations of workplace stress qualify as work-related.
- Stress is not always a bad thing.
- An individual can tolerate a brief exposure to stress, which may be beneficial.
- No exhaustive list of potential stress indicators is provided.
- Certain "symptoms" (frequent absenteeism, interpersonal conflict, etc.) point to the presence of work-related stress.
- A problem can be pinpointed by analyzing factors such as organizational arrangements, workplace conditions and environments, the effectiveness of communications and subjective factors.
- Once a problem relating to stress has been identified, action must be taken to prevent, eliminate or reduce it.
- The responsibility for establishing appropriate measures lies with the employer, who can integrate the measures into the risk assessment process and put them into effect with the collaboration of the workers and/or their representatives.
- Measurements can be collective, individual or a mixture of both.
- Use can be made of outside experts.

In Italy, the European Agreement was adopted a few months after the enactment of Legislative Decree 81/08 with the signing of the Interconfederal Agreement of June 9, 2008 (Confindustria et al., 2008).

The 2004 Agreement therefore forms the legal–methodological basis for the assessment of work-related stress ("work stress") in Europe. The Agreement was first included as a binding reference document for employers by Article 28 of Legislative Decree 81/08 and was subsequently adopted in Italy when trade unions signed the Interconfederal Agreement of 2008. Pursuant to Article 6.8 of the same Legislative Decree, the Advisory Committee of the Italian Ministry of Labor issued guidelines on the operating methodologies to be followed as a matter of obligation. The Advisory Committee thus mandated a set of minimum operating methodologies that employers must observe when conducting risk assessments and established the obligation for employers always to carry out a "preliminary" assessment, to be succeeded, only where necessary, by an "in-depth" assessment.

The preliminary assessment consists in identifying indicators that are objective, verifiable and, preferably, expressible in numerical terms. For the purpose of identifying these indicators, employers should be mindful of the following aspects of the methodology:

- Evaluating the risk of stress in the workplace is an integral part of the more general risk assessment process (Article 28/81).
- The evaluation shall be carried out by the employer, who shall deputize the task to the Occupational Health and Safety Officer (OHSO) and, where present, to the Occupational Health Physician (OHP), and shall also take advice from the workers' Occupational Health and Safety Representative (OHSR).
- The assessment refers to **all** workers (including managers and supervisors).

- Assessments are not conducted on individual workers, rather they must be conducted on **homogeneous groups of workers**, as identified by the employer.
- The assessment consists of two phases:
  a. Preliminary (always compulsory);
  b. In-depth (required only if risks have been detected in the preceding phase).
- The preliminary assessment consists in identifying objective, verifiable and, where possible, numerically expressible indicators that belong to at least three distinct families:
  I. Sentinel events;
  II. Work content factors;
  III. Work context factors.
- An assessment of the content and context of work (as per points II and III above) must also involve **listening to the views of the workers** and/or their health and safety representative(s) (OHSR). Larger companies may use a representative sample of workers for this purpose. **Employers are free to choose the specific means by which they will listen to the opinions of workers, which will depend also on the assessment methodology they are using.**
- If the preliminary assessment does not result in the discovery of any risks from work-related stress that would necessitate corrective action, then the employer shall be required only to note the findings in the Risk Assessment Document and to draw up a risk-monitoring plan.
- (…)If the assessment does result in the discovery of risks from work stress requiring corrective action, then the employer shall plan and implement appropriate corrective actions. If the corrective actions should prove ineffective, then the next step (…) is to carry out an **"in-depth" risk assessment**. An in-depth assessment entails taking stock of the subjective perception of workers regarding the abovementioned stress–risk factors/families of indicators through the use of various survey tools, such as, for example, questionnaires, focus groups and semi-structured interviews.

2.3.2 INDICATORS USED IN THE PRELIMINARY ASSESSMENT

The three families of "objective and verifiable" indicators on which the preliminary assessment should be based are, by and large, the following:

I. *Sentinel events:* accident rates; the number of sick leaves; worker turnover; procedures, sanctions and reports issued by the occupational health physician (OHP); specific and frequent formal complaints submitted by workers.
II. *Content factors:* the working environment and equipment, workloads and rhythms, working hours and shifts, the consonance of workers' skills with the professional duties they are expected to perform.
III. *Context factors:* the worker's organizational function, decision-making autonomy and control, the presence of interpersonal conflicts in the working environment, career development and advancement, communication issues (e.g. uncertainty surrounding what is being asked of the worker).

It is more accurate to consider "sentinel events" as the first actual "**signs of harm**" rather than simply as indicators of potential risk, for they may, in fact, be the tangible and objective consequences of stressful situations that are not being properly dealt with in the workplace. As such, they need to be addressed and mediated through the preliminary assessment process described below. Likewise, while the workers' OHSR must necessarily be consulted, the workers themselves (to be treated collectively as members of a homogeneous group rather than individually) must also be listened to, including at the preliminary assessment phase, for the proper way to understand the workplace context is to view it as being: *a "collective" arrangement,* an interpretation that adheres most closely to the recommendations and spirit of the European Agreement, which declares that:

- Work-related stress can be caused by various factors, such as the content and organization of work, the working environment, poor communications, etc.
- Given the complexity of the stress phenomenon, this Agreement does not intend to provide an exhaustive list of potential stress indicators. However, high absenteeism or staff turnover, frequent interpersonal conflicts or complaints by workers are some of the signs that may indicate a problem of work-related stress.
- Identifying whether there is a problem of work-related stress can involve an analysis of factors such as work organization and processes (working time arrangements, degree of autonomy, match between workers skills and job requirements, workload, etc.), working conditions and environment (exposure to abusive behavior, noise, heat, dangerous substances, etc.), communication (uncertainty about what is expected at work, employment prospects, or forthcoming change, etc.) and subjective factors (emotional and social pressures, feeling unable to cope, perceived lack of support, etc.).

2.3.3 PARTICIPATION OF WORKERS AND HOMOGENEOUS GROUPS

Worker participation is fundamental, including at the preliminary phase, because:

Workers are '**privileged observers**' of the employing entity, because they are part of it and have direct experience of it in their lives. The risks associated with workplace stress can be traced back to two mutually interacting areas: the potential of the work itself to induce stress and workers' perception of their ability to adapt themselves to the working conditions. It follows that the only way to evaluate work context and work content factors is by involving the workers. For their involvement to be effective, workers need to be adequately apprised of the nature of the risk, of the negative effects of stress on individual workers and on the company organization, and of the evaluation methodology being used.

Worker participation is necessary both at the preliminary and at the in-depth phase, though the form of participation will vary according to which phase is in play. **At the preliminary phase, "observational" checklists (i.e. based on a list of observations concerning issues in need of attention) cannot be considered reliable unless workers and/or their OHSR have been involved in their preparation**.

Similarly, the methodological approach being proposed here conforms to the directives governing the succession of phases and the rules for their implementation as given in a 2012 document produced by the Committee Interregional for Prevention (CIP) (Coordinamento Tecnico Interregionale della Prevenzione nei Luoghi di Lavoro, 2012).

The following indications, here reproduced in full, dictated the framing of the questions and responses and the manner in which the checklist was administered to the homogeneous group of workers:

- Sentinel events are those of which the employing company has already taken note for other purposes. Context and content factors, on the other hand, are evaluated by means of a specifically observation-based analysis. Where a checklist of context and content factors is compiled, the results that it produces derive not from subjective perceptions of stress factors but from an appraisal of the organizational effectiveness of the workplace at mitigating and countering the negative aspects of these factors, which are therefore included as items in the checklist.
- The checklist items that necessitate further investigation are those pertaining to the work context and content, and to sentinel events, which, as is the norm with most of the applicable methods, need to be evaluated from a holistic perspective.

A key moment in the process is when the homogeneous group of workers within the company organization is identified and selected. The methods for selecting which workers will be associated with which homogenous group are set out in precise detail in the aforementioned CIP document:

- Given that the purpose of the evaluation is to identify and apply corrective measures, the analysis, in addition to flagging up issues in need of attention, must also clearly indicate which jobs and which groups of workers are affected by them. If the analytical methodology consists of collating observations gathered at a collective level, as is done when compiling a checklist, then the subdivision of workers into homogeneous groups or their designation to separate divisions in the organization must be carried out in advance, during the risk-assessment planning phase. When designating workers to a given homogeneous group, it is important to ensure that the designation criteria correspond to the actual organizational arrangements of the company. The reason for this is that proper categorization will facilitate the task of analyzing the sentinel events and the content and context factors that are specific to the designated homogenous group and will reveal the extent to which various stress factors are ascribable to different situations within the company.
- The division of workers into groups should reflect both how the company actually apportions the work among its employees and how it operates in a specific territorial context.
- Companies that are organizationally less complex (i.e. those with 30 or fewer employees) may proceed with preliminary assessments without having first to identify separate organizational segments or homogeneous groups. Such companies do not need to set up separate areas of operations

because their workers share the working environment, use the same model of communication and report directly to company management. As a rule, there is little point in dividing workers into homogenous groups if the division, whether based on activities or job assignment, is inconsequential for the purposes of the stress–risk assessment (e.g. if a company is made up of two managers, two sales representatives, three logistics operators and six manual workers) or if the particular conditions of individual workers are such that it is impossible accurately to assess or prevent work-related stress.

- Larger companies, by contrast, must carry out assessments that befit the complexity of their organizational structures and must therefore decide whether to divide their workforce along the same lines as internal company departments or to assign them to homogenous groups, or both. Assigning workers to homogeneous groups that correspond to actual corporate structures ensures the establishment of a sound process of preliminary assessment, facilitates the adoption of any necessary corrective actions and the verification of their effectiveness and creates the conditions for the possible activation of an in-depth assessment.
- The identification of homogeneous groups is the responsibility of management, which shall work with the OHSO, the OHP (where appointed) and the OHSR to this end. Various criteria may be used for the designation of homogenous groups, such as:
  - Categorization based on type of activity (offices, structures, departments);
  - Categorization based on type of job assignment;
  - Categorization based on level of exposure to known risks (e.g. call centers, dealing with distressed customers/users, etc.);
  - Categorization based on type of employment contract.
- A decision not to designate workers to homogeneous groups needs to be justified and must also be consistent with the organizational arrangements of the company. Generally speaking, it is not advisable to assign employees who work in different locations to the same homogenous group, unless the workers in question are exposed to the same type of risks. Our experience suggests that 2–3 groups of workers should be listened to for every 100 workers identified as belonging to a homogeneous group in accordance with the foregoing criteria.

In conclusion, the step-by-step procedures for assessing work-related stress are encapsulated in the standards and good practices mentioned above, and the observational checklist proposed here faithfully reproduces each of these steps, which are summarized below:

- The assessment of the risk of work-related stress is part and parcel of a broader assessment of occupational health and safety that employers are required to perform pursuant to, with respect to the specific risk of stress, the European Framework Agreement of 2004.
- Employers are free to choose the methodology they consider most appropriate for their company, but the methodology must be consistent with the

recommendations of the European Framework Agreement transposed into Italian law, and the instructions of the CIP, all of which constitute "good practices" under the meaning of Article 2/81.

- The assessment is mandatory for all companies, whether in the private or the public sector and for all workers, including managers and supervisors.
- At all phases of the process, due heed must be paid to the views of the OHSR and the workers, who, on the basis of pre-established and declared criteria, shall have been designated to the appropriate homogeneous group. If identifying a homogeneous group is objectively impossible, an explicit declaration to this effect must be made.
- The object of the assessment is to estimate the extent of the presumed damage: it is not to determine the exact extent of the damage to the workers themselves, as this is the job of the company doctor (OHP), who works with qualified experts to this end.
- The preliminary assessment is mandatory for all companies. Depending on the results of the preliminary assessment, it may or may not be followed by an in-depth assessment.
- The preliminary assessment must consider three families of factors (sentinel events, work content and work context), all of which need to be examined in full.
- Even if the assessment results in favorable reports, a periodic risk-monitoring plan must nonetheless be prepared.

2.3.4 SCIENTIFIC REFERENCE SOURCES ON WORK-RELATED STRESS

Work-related stress is a complex issue that does not admit of easy definition or evaluation. Consequently, even though it is one of the commonest forms of risk exposure for workers in Europe, it is a difficult phenomenon to measure.

A brief review of the most important scientific reference sources dealing with work stress is therefore in order and should help dispel a number of prejudices and myths. Indeed, some of the misunderstandings arise not only from the way in which the term "stress" is used in everyday language but also from its use in technical–scientific literature.

In common parlance, "stress" is something of a catch-all term that can signify several different things, all of them relating in some way to the idea that humans respond and adapt in certain ways to changes in their physical or psychosocial environment. Its indiscriminate use in everyday language means that "stressful" or "stressed" may be used to denote the attitude or character of a person, to describe a situation (e.g. an environment may also be described as "stressful"), or to characterize the state of mind of a person in relation to an event (e.g. "I am feeling very stressed"). Even when the term is used in a scientific context, its definition remains loose. Jex et al. (Jex, 1992) carried out a survey of how the term is used in the six major scientific journals (from 1985 to 1989) dedicated to organizational behavior. The researchers found that 41% of the 51 articles they examined used the word "stress" to denote the stimulus that triggered the stress reaction, 22% used it to denote the reaction itself and 25% used it in reference to both the stimulus and the reaction.

The peculiar characteristics of work-related stress, characteristics that differentiate it from other dangers, are also part of what makes it so complex a concept. The first distinguishing peculiarity is that the term refers to intangible sources of danger. Whereas a physical–ergonomic danger has a concrete and visible source, stress refers to a danger whose source is not materially identifiable but is to be found instead in how the human mind apprehends the complex nature of reality.

A second distinguishing peculiarity has to do with how a risk/danger has consequences for a person's health. While a physical risk and the potential of that risk to cause harm can be mapped to organs of the human body whose structures are for the most part known and whose functions are essentially amenable to mechanical description (e.g. how noise affects the ear and can cause hearing loss, or how the strain of lifting affects the muscles and can cause lower back pain), the effects of stress on human health have to be measured with reference to a human organ whose workings are still the subject of study and whose functions are not as amenable to mechanical description, namely the human mind.

These two peculiarities alone are sufficient justification for affirming that stress in the workplace is the most complex type of risk to which workers are exposed.

The complexities of the phenomenon notwithstanding, the scientific study of stress for more than a century has led to the establishment of a number of certainties.

The first scientific studies into stress date back to the early years of the last century. The studies were mainly interested in physiological reactions to conditions of stress. At the time, the word "stress" was mostly used in the field of engineering, where it referred to the source of danger or the cause of a condition of stress.

Walter Cannon (Cannon, 1929, 1932), an American physiologist, was one of the first researchers to examine how creatures react to stress. It was Cannon who identified what he termed the "fight-or-flight response", which refers to the physiological changes that a living being undergoes in order to protect against an external threat. He identified the reaction as originating in the limbic system of the brain, while much more recent studies have stipulated that the reaction actually originates in the amygdala, which is a gland to be found in the limbic system (Rodrigues et al., 2009). Specifically, Cannon described the "physiological cascade" that occurs when the fight-or-flight response is triggered in the face of a perceived threat. The main consequences of the activation of the fight-or-flight response are shown in Figure 2.13.

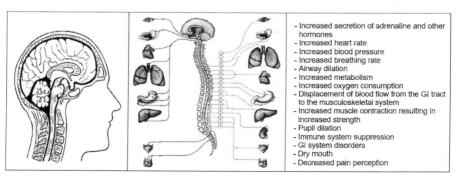

- Increased secretion of adrenaline and other hormones
- Increased heart rate
- Increased blood pressure
- Increased breathing rate
- Airway dilation
- Increased metabolism
- Increased oxygen consumption
- Displacement of blood flow from the GI tract to the musculoskeletal system
- Increased muscle contraction resulting in increased strength
- Pupil dilation
- Immune system suppression
- GI system disorders
- Dry mouth
- Decreased pain perception

FIGURE 2.13 Main physiological changes triggered by a threat (fight-or-flight response).

All the changes brought about by the triggering of our fight-or-flight response work towards enhancing our physical performance so that we are better prepared and quicker to enter into the fight-or-flight mode when our survival is at stake. In this respect, reactivity to stress enables us to face threats and create conditions favorable for our survival and is a normal feature of everyday life. When the stress response is transient and not excessively intense, it is unquestionably beneficial. Indeed, only in death is stress entirely absent, in that we become completely stress-free only when we stop interacting in any way with the external environment.

Usually, however, the term stress is used in reference to the negative repercussions of this life-saving function, which occur either when the response is too intense (traumatic stress) or when the stress, albeit at a lower intensity, occurs too frequently or lasts for too prolonged a period (this is known as chronic stress, and is typical of work-related stress).

Hans Selye, a physician with clinical experience, identified the negative effects of exposure to chronic stress (Selye, 1936, 1974), and advanced the theory of what he called the General Adaptation Syndrome. He posited that a stress response could be divided into three consecutive stages (Figure 2.14). The first is the "alarm reaction stage", which is similar to the fight-or-flight response mentioned above. If the stressor – the original stimulus that triggered the fight-or-flight response – persists, then the second "resistance stage" comes into play, during which the organism seeks to counter any recurrence of the stress response. During this stage, the body experiences short-term reactions with which we are all familiar appear: stomach pain, difficulty sleeping, anxiety, etc. The third and final "exhaustion stage" takes over if the resistance stage is so prolonged that it depletes the body's energy and the sufferer becomes incapable of continuing to

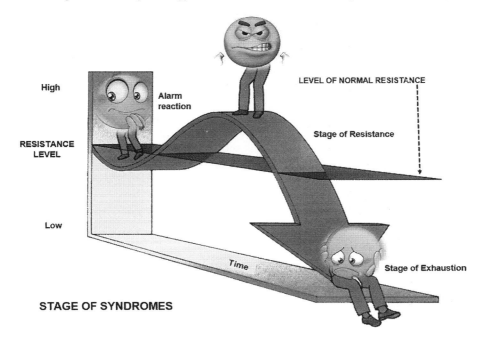

FIGURE 2.14 Response to prolonged stress (Selye, 1936, 1974).

resist the state of stress. An individual at the exhaustion stage will experience conditions of stress in a way that is very harmful to his or her health.

Selye's research popularized the term stress, and gave currency to the idea that stress referred to the negative reaction induced by the presence of a difficulty or threat.

Stress studies continued with Richard Lazarus, an interpreter of cognitive sciences, who accounted for the variability of individual stress responses by introducing the concept of the "cognitive filter", which explains how individuals may have different perceptions of stress even when the stressor is the same (Lazarus, 1966). The cognitive filter is the mental process by which different persons attribute different meanings to their experience of reality. Lazarus's theory explains why different people respond with different stress levels to the same stressful event. In Lazarus's paradigm, stress is defined as the change that occurs in the condition of the organism in response to a stressor.

European regulations in this area have taken on board all the latest scientific findings, and the European Framework Agreement on work-related stress therefore defines it as being "a state which is accompanied by physical, psychological or social complaints or dysfunctions and which results from individuals feeling unable to meet the requirements or expectations placed on them".

This definition identifies stress as "a state" rather than as a stimulus or psycho-physiological response, though it also encompasses both these latter connotations. Accordingly, the term "stress" is used to refer to working conditions that have negative repercussions on the health of the worker.

Another interesting distinction can be made between the generic term "stress" and the more specific term "work-related stress". While the generic term refers to a natural condition that accompanies us throughout our lives, "work stress" (or "work-related stress") is a condition that excludes all the positive aspects of stress and is comprised solely of its negative aspects, such as biopsychosocial illness and dysfunction.

Finally, the reference in the foregoing definition to "individuals feeling unable to meet" what is asked of them relates the concept of workplace stress to working conditions. The definition therefore incorporates Lazarus's findings and relates stress to the way in which external stimuli affect how humans function. The significance of this last point should not be misconstrued. Whereas individual perception is certainly one of the elements of stress, this should not be taken as meaning that the level of work stress depends entirely on the individual person. Figure 2.15 shows an example of how a stressful condition can lead to the onset of a pathology.

The research that followed Lazarus has established, with particular regard to work-related stress, that certain working conditions have an impact on occupational health. i.e., on the health of most workers.

Research over the last 30 years into the effects of work stress on human health has explored the connections between certain working conditions and the health of the working population. The literature on the subject includes, to cite just a few examples, Netterstrøm et al., 2008 (on the depressive effects of work stress); Stansfeld and Candy, 2006 (on psychological health); Kivimäki et al., 2006 and 2012 (on physical health); and Linton et al., 2015 (on sleep disturbances).

Researchers have always tried to reduce the complexity of the phenomenon of work-related stress by producing schematic models. The models, which are

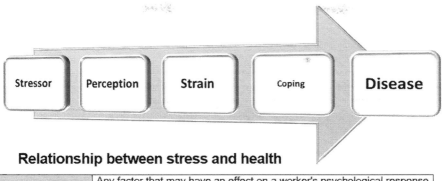

Relationship between stress and health

STRESSOR	Any factor that may have an effect on a worker's psychological response to his or her work or working conditions (including relations with his or her superiors and co-workers)
PERCEPTION	Cognitive and emotional evaluation ("cognitive filter")
STRAIN	Short-term physical, emotional and cognitive manifestations due to physiological activation
COPING	Activities put in place to resist stress
DISEASE	Pathological health and social consequences

FIGURE 2.15 Simplified depiction of the relationship between stress and sickness.

simplifications of a complex phenomenon, seek to describe the relationships between the principal factors of stress and have been validated through scientific research.

The best-known stress models are Karasek's Job Demands Control Support (Karasek et al., 1990), which predicates three key determinants of work stress:

1. Job demand (the size of the workload);
2. Job decision-making latitude (the autonomy enjoyed by the employee to use his or her skills);
3. Quality of social support from co-workers and superiors.

Siegrist's Effort Reward Imbalance model (Siegrist et al., 2004) presupposes a condition of negative stress whenever there is an imbalance between the efforts that the worker puts into the work and the rewards (which are not only material) that he or she receives from the same.

The Job Demands Resources or JD-R model (Bakker and Demerouti, 2007, 2017) has been one of the most extensively studied in recent years. It is the newest of the working models for the evaluation of work-related stress, and is used as the reference standard for the production of Quick Assessments.

The JD-R and the studies associated with it introduced some new points that had not been included in the earlier models, namely:

1. The psychosocial setting of the workplace is determined by the balance of demands and resources. Demands are all those aspects of a job that have a psychophysical cost on the worker; the resources are all those elements that are conducive to the achievement by that worker of his or her work objectives, and that support the worker's personal and professional growth.

2. The most innovative element of this model is that it divides the demands and resources into two different processes: the former impact directly on the worker's health and the latter on the worker's motivation and job satisfaction.

This model (Figure 2.16) has provided the guidelines for compiling the risk pre-mapping document, the purpose of which is to accord the highest prominence to stressors with the greatest impact on the health of workers, but to consider them separately from the elements contributing to worker motivation, which are also taken into consideration, albeit to a more limited extent.

As noted earlier, work-related stress is a state "accompanied by physical, psychological or social complaints or dysfunctions"; in other words, it impacts workers' health, not their (de)motivation. For this reason, an assessment of the risk of work-related stress cannot be chiefly based on a collation of workers' complaints and expressions of dissatisfaction, but must be based instead on an analysis of working conditions, for its real purpose is to detect possible instances of working conditions that are known to be harmful to a majority of workers.

The JD-R model is capable of giving full account of every condition with the potential to impact health and motivation, but of all the conditions that are considered in an evaluation, pre-eminence must be given to the quadrant labelled "strain" (see figure), which refers to all conditions and factors with a potential impact on workers' health. This quadrant is directly connected with "Job Demands"

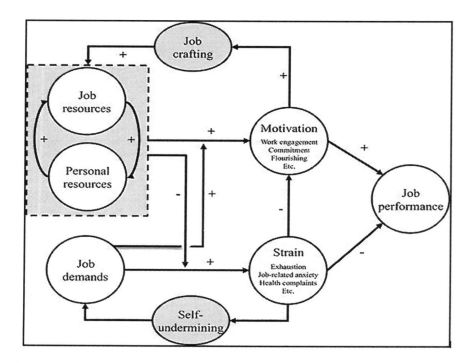

FIGURE 2.16   Job Demand-Resources Model (Bakker and Demerouti, 2017).

(see figure), which thus become the most salient elements in the evaluation. By con-trast, although Job Resources (see figure) directly impact on motivation, they have a moderating effect on the relationship between work demands and health; that is to say, Job Resources regulate the relationship and can cushion or amplify final effects on health. Job Resources therefore prove their worth when they can be used to support major work demands.

In order to determine which Job Resources and which Job Demands need to be included in the evaluation, reference has been made to the vast volume of research on the connection between work stress and health. The aim is to identify which fac-tors recur most often and how consequential they are for worker health. The factors considered include those that, as the research papers note, play a large role in the engendering of stressful working conditions. The factors that were also identified by the other models described above are workload, pace of work, emotional com-mitment, etc. Other factors (such as home-work conflict or an uncomfortable work environment) were found to be of more limited application.

The assessment document takes into account the latest scientific thinking on the subject and presents it in a simplified and streamlined manner. It takes full account of the largest constituent elements of the phenomenon and defines them objectively with the aim of reaching an initial general assessment that shares features with a Quick Assessment performed using the ERGOCHECK tool.

The solid scientific relevance of the resulting data notwithstanding, the assess-ment document is not intended to be used as part of a broad-ranging review of work stress in general. Rather, it is intended only for the purposes of producing a simple, quick, first determination of whether or not factors potentially detrimental to health are present in the working activity under review, or whether there is a risk to health.

In practice, even if work stress is measured on a spectrum ranging from motivation/involvement to pathology, this part of the Quick Assessment is useful for detecting the presence of work place discomfort that requires corrective action (if potential solutions are near to hand) or else the carrying out of an in-depth assessment that uses different methodologies.

Motivation, which lies on the opposite side of stress, is also registered in the course of the survey (spontaneous statements made about motivational factors can be noted down) but is not one of the factors considered when defining stress exposure metrics. The focus remains narrowly angled towards a specific part of the reference model, namely the part referring to health.

3 Pre-mapping of Risk Factors for Occupational Health and Wellbeing
General Structure of ERGOCHECK

Daniela Colombini and Enrico Occhipinti
Ergonomics of Posture and Movements
International Ergonomics School (EPM-IES)

CONTENTS

3.1 INTRODUCTION

As stated previously, one of the latest developments being pursued by the World Health Organization (WHO) and other international organizations (ILO, ISO), in relation to preventing work-related diseases and disorders, concerns the creation of simplified toolkits that can also be used by non-experts in occupational health and industrial hygiene.

The main aim is to rapidly but accurately identify the presence of possible sources of risk, using tools that can easily be used by Occupational Health and Safety (OSH) operators, occupational physicians, employers, workers, trade union representatives and labor inspector officers.

However, this objective also reflects the criteria set forth in ISO/TR 12295 (ISO, 2014) with respect to the risk of biomechanical overload, as mentioned above.

Against this backdrop, and for preventive purposes, the problems that give rise to WMSDs should be considered along with other occupational hazards (physical, chemical, organizational, etc.) (Colombini and Occhipinti, 2011; Occhipinti and Colombini, 2016).

This book suggests a methodology and some simple tools for adopting a participatory approach toward exposed workers in order to undertake a *preliminary mapping of discomfort/hazards* in the workplace (i.e. to identify risk sources in the job cycle), especially in small and very small businesses.

The tool does not pretend to replace the standard risk assessment process, but to support such a process so as to identify hazardous situations in the workplace, based on which to determine emerging problems that need to be submitted to a full risk assessment based on priorities (i.e. analytical evaluations and/or risk reduction).

As well, the tool can be used by employers and/or trade union representatives to more readily identify situations that may also call for the involvement of an occupational health expert to be present during the assessment.

3.2 GENERAL PRE-MAPPING MODEL UTILIZING ERGOCHECK

The operation involves two levels of analysis and intervention.

The first level entails a rapid and general identification of possible sources of risk via the use of specific *key enters*. This preliminary level ensures that all users (regardless of their skills and education) can simply and generally observe the overall workplace. The first level can be broken down into several "sections" based on the main types of risks: *manual load handling, repetitive movements of the upper limbs, postures, noise, microclimate, vibrations, equipment/tools, chemical/biological agents, stress, etc.*

It should be emphasized that with regard to biomechanical overload and chemical, physical and biological agents, the first level consists of actual *key enters* that may or may not require the completion of specific second-level worksheets (*quick assessment*). Conversely, for all the other risk factors (microclimate, noise, vibrations, etc.) the first-level phase overlaps with the second-level phase in the model (*key questions = combination of key enters + quick assessment*).

In the *second-level phase* (*quick assessment*) the level attention that needs to be focussed on a certain risk factor is estimated. From time to time, this estimate may identify definitely exposure conditions as acceptable (indicated using the traditional traffic light system, as *code green*), definitely very high (*code critical*, or *purple*) or even intermediate, between the previous two, which in turn may be acceptable, borderline, significant or very high. This applies to all aspects relating to biomechanical overload (lifting and carrying, pushing and pulling, repetitive movements of the upper limbs, awkward postures of the whole body) and chemical, physical and biological agents, as well as to the fundamental aspect of stress (work-related), for which the initial phase of the *key enters* was not planned.

If the situation is *code green* the risk assessment process could even stop here because it means that there is no meaningful occupational risk.

If a *code critical* situation is detected, then there is definitely a significant occupational risk and immediate corrective actions are required.

If the quick assessment finds that the risk level at the work station is neither acceptable (*green*) nor critical (*purple*), and therefore, that the situation is intermediate (potentially *code yellow, red*, or even *purple*), then the risk assessment will have to be carried out using the analytical methods (generally first level – risk estimate) suggested by ISO standards or the accredited literature; it may be necessary to put corrective actions in place to directly remedy the most problematic conditions.

The pre-mapping phase never calls for instrumental measurements and must be undertaken by consulting with the *homogeneous group of workers*.

Here *homogeneous group* refers to a group of workers performing the same task or set of tasks in the same place, for the same duration and with the same exposure conditions.

The worksheet is therefore not completed with reference to the company, department or (generic) task, but takes into account the organizational set-up in the workplace under examination for groups of workers who are homogeneous in terms of exposure.

The homogeneous group may occasionally be comprised of only one person, but it is more common for the homogeneous group to include several workers assigned to various processes or workstations, which must obviously be identical also in terms of duration for all the workers belonging to the same group, as often is the case in small companies.

Similarly, the homogeneous group may even be fairly large, in which case the opinions and modal judgments of the group will be taken into account; in yet other cases the homogeneous group may consist of one person; therefore, the opinions of that individual worker will be considered.

To fill in the worksheet, the examiner meets and interviews the homogeneous group. As the answers entered into the worksheet will be based on their opinions, the examiner may occasionally find it necessary to encourage discussions, particularly when there are differences of opinion within the group. In any case, the examiner cannot substitute his or her opinions for those expressed by the homogeneous group.

The preliminary mapping methodology consists in an easy-to-use computer-based model (ERGOCHECK) for collecting data (Excel spreadsheet: **epmiesERGOCHECKpremapGLOBeng**), available for free download in Italian or English from *www.epmresearch.org*.

The model consists of several pages (worksheets) with closed-ended questions that in most cases requires placing a cross on the appropriate answer, and in only a few cases, calls for simple numbers to be entered.

Once all the various sections of the worksheet have been completed, the software automatically displays information about the priority level for the risk factor considered, usually in the form of traffic lights and/or colors. The colors may be *green* (problem absent or negligible), *yellow* (problem present but minor), *red* (problem present, requires further analysis), *purple* (problem present, situation definitely critical, urgent action or in-depth analysis required). Since the pre-mapping exercise aims to set priorities for each individual risk factor examined, it was a deliberate decision to avoid assigning a score to these initial indicators, and rather to use colors to depict either the absence of the problem or the presence of the problem and the need to deal with it more or less urgently (color-coded priorities). The worksheets presenting the conclusions of the quick assessment of a given risk factor indicate colors along with short comments on priority levels and consequent corrective actions.

Priority levels are based on ordinal (arbitrary) scales of scores (not visible but useful for processing) that rise as each risk factor moves from fully acceptable conditions (minimum score) to clearly critical situations (maximum score), adjusting the scores for intermediate conditions.

Intermediate scores are usually compared with the maximum score indicated, and the relevant fraction (or percentage) is used to express priority as a color.

Generally speaking, and with minor variations with respect to the various risk factors, the quick assessment worksheets and final summary indicate:

- Priority *green* (acceptable risk): up to 30% of maximum;
- Priority *yellow* (probable slight or very slight risk): up to 50% of maximum;
- Priority *red* (probable risk present): between 50% and 80% of maximum;
- Priority *purple* (probable very high or critical risk): more than 80% of maximum.

These scores should not be regarded as "predictors of the likelihood of disease": they are merely "indicators" of greater or lesser levels of exposure to risk.

4 First-Level Pre-mapping
Key Enters and General Overview

Daniela Colombini and Enrico Occhipinti
Ergonomics of Posture and Movements
International Ergonomics School (EPM-IES)

CONTENTS

The ERGOCHECK software is comprised of Excel work sheets, and the first pre-mapping level involves inserting the necessary key enters (Figure 4.1).

The first section is comprised of several parts (boxes) devoted to the various risk factors and includes preliminary data concerning the workers.

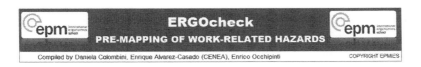

FIGURE 4.1   ERGOCHECK – Front page of the general overview.

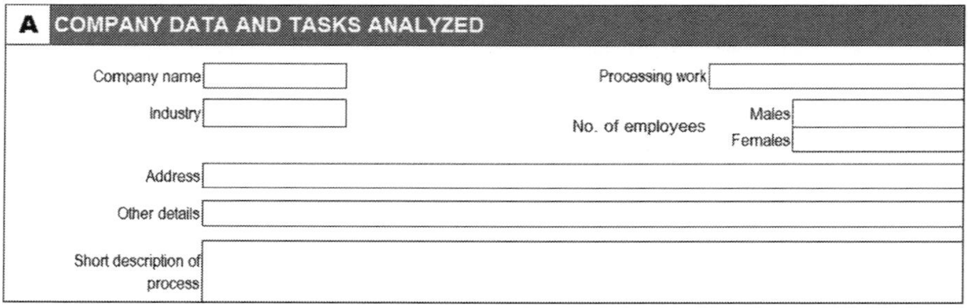

A COMPANY DATA AND TASKS ANALYZED

Company name

Industry

Processing work

No. of employees: Males / Females

Address

Other details

Short description of process

FIGURE 4.2 Data concerning the company and description of the homogeneous group.

4.1 DATA CONCERNING THE COMPANY AND THE HOMOGENEOUS GROUP

Once the facility has been described, the pre-mapping work sheet is completed for an individual worker or group of workers (homogeneous group) who perform the same task(s) the same way and with the same exposure time. The term "job" is used to describe a set of tasks performed in a typical shift or longer time frame. In this case, it is useful to describe the working period during which the homogeneous group is exposed to risk, for instance, a representative month of the year, or even an entire year, within which workers are rotated between different tasks. A separate pre-mapping work sheet must be used for each homogeneous group of workers (Figure 4.2).

4.2 KEY ENTERS FOR PRIORITIZING THE EVALUATION OF BIOMECHANICAL OVERLOAD

The various biomechanical risks are then identified in terms of presence or absence, using the same key enters as those proposed in ISO/TR 12295 (Figures 4.3 and 4.4). The key enters are actually very simple questions with YES/NO answers that reveal whether potential sources of risk (e.g. load lifting) in a certain process need further evaluation. Depending on the situation, there may be no load lifting risk because the object weighs less than 3 kg, or, if the object to be lifted weighs 3 kg or more, then task will need analyzing.

These key enters allow anyone analyzing occupational risk exposure to quickly and unequivocally know whether or not further assessments are required.

Figure 4.3 (depicting the Excel spreadsheet) indicates the corresponding key enters for determining whether repetitive movements, lifting, moving and pushing and pulling tasks require evaluation. The spreadsheets include a few "HELPS" to decide whether or not a more in-depth analysis is required.

As far as biomechanical overload due to awkward postures is concerned, particularly of the spine and lower limbs, reference is made to the key enter indicated by ISO/TR 12295 but using a simpler and more comprehensible version

B	**BIOMECHANICAL OVERLOAD**		

B1	**BIOMECHANICAL OVERLOAD OF UPPER LIMBS IN REPETITIVE TASKS**

PRESENCE OF REPETITIVE TASKS: The task is organized in cycles, regardless of their duration, or the task is characterized by similar working gestures for over 50% of the time. The term "repetitive" does not mean risk is present. **YES** / **NO**

B2	**BIOMECHANICAL OVERLOAD FROM MANUAL HANDLING - LIFTING**

PRESENCE OF OBJECTS WEIGHING 3 KG OR MORE TO BE MANUALLY LIFTED (if the weight is less, no need to continue the investigation) **YES** / **NO**

B3	**BIOMECHANICAL OVERLOAD FROM MANUAL HANDLING - CARRYING**

PRESENCE OF OBJECTS EXCEEDING 3 KG TO BE MANUALLY CARRIED (if the loads are lighter, there is no need to continue the investigation). **YES** / **NO**

B4	**BIOMECHANICAL OVERLOAD FROM MANUAL PUSHING AND PULLING**

IS THERE WHOLE-BODY PUSHING OR PULLING OF LOADS? **YES** / **NO**

FIGURE 4.3 Key enters for defining assessment priorities in relation to biomechanical overload due to repetitive movements of the upper limbs and manual load handling.

B6	**BIOMECHANICAL OVERLOAD FROM AWKWARD POSTURES - TRUNK AND LOWER LIMBS**

Are there static or awkward working postures of the HEAD/NECK, TRUNK and/or UPPER AND LOWER LIMBS maintained for more than 4 seconds consecutively and repeated for a significant proportion of the working time? **YES**

In practice, in general, postures are not awkward (INDICATE "NO") when the subject: **NO**
- is sitting with the back well supported, adequate leg room and can stand up (change position) at least every hour.
- is standing with the trunk erect (no deep bending or twisting) but free to walk around or sit at least every hour (with the back well supported and adequate leg room).

i.e. If YES, please specify for which segment there are awkward postures | **NO** | **YES** |

HEAD/NECK (neck bent back/forward/sideways, twisted)

TRUNK (trunk bent forward/sideways/, back bent with no support, twisted)

UPPER LIMBS (hand(s) at or above head, elbow(s) at or above shoulder level, elbow/hand(s) behind the body, hand(s) turned with palms completely up or down, extreme elbow flexion-extension, wrist bent forward/back/sideways)

LOWER LIMBS (squatting or kneeling) with position maintained for more than 4 seconds consecutively and repeated for a significant proportion of the working time

FIGURE 4.4 Key enters for defining assessment priorities in relation to working posture.

(Figure 4.4). In other words, awkward postures do not need to be further examined if the worker:

- Is sitting with back well supported, has enough leg room and can get up and change position at least every hour.
- Is standing up straight (without bending or twisting the upper body) but able to move around or sit down at least every hour (with back well supported and enough leg room).

To help compile this initial description of postures, a few figures have been provided to illustrate the most common awkward working postures. The questions only require a YES or NO answer to indicate the presence or absence of the posture.

If any of the conditions indicated as awkward are present, it will be necessary to examine postures in greater detail in the subsequent *quick assessment* work sheet (see Section 5.5), with distinctions being made as to whether the awkward postures concern the upper limbs (quick assessment of repetitive upper limb movements) and/or the spine and/or lower limbs (quick assessment of working postures).

For all conditions of exposure to biomechanical overload, once the presence of the event has been evidenced (positive key enters), the next step is to complete the specific quick assessment work sheets (second evaluation phase).

4.3 KEY QUESTIONS FOR IDENTIFYING LIGHTING PROBLEMS

As for all the other sections of the pre-mapping work sheet, these questions are also closed-ended and refer to the visual effort required to perform the work in relation to the lighting both at the work station and in the work place in general, and to the work surfaces and surfaces of the objects being worked (Figure 4.5).

It is advisable to ask these questions by interviewing the members of the homogeneous group; each one should be asked to express their opinion regarding the type of lighting, i.e. whether it is sufficient, poor or excessive, also in relation to the time frame, in other words: *for a few hours a day or all day.* The workers are also asked about the surfaces of their work benches and of the objects being handled, i.e., whether they are opaque or shiny.

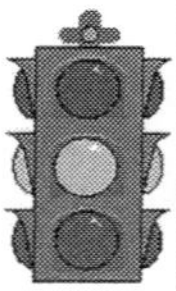

FIGURE 4.5 Key questions for identifying indoor (and outdoor) lighting issues.

4.4 KEY QUESTIONS FOR IDENTIFYING ISSUES DUE TO EXPOSURE TO UV RADIATION (SOLAR OR WELDING)

With regard to detecting the possible existence of a problem due to exposure to solar ultraviolet (UV) radiation, all that is considered here is the time spent working out of doors (Figure 4.6).

With reference to welding, the analysis asks whether the work involves low, medium or high exposure to UV radiation. A description of the type of work needs adding in the notes, along with the type of welding process and presence or absence of protective gear.

4.5 KEY QUESTIONS FOR IDENTIFYING ISSUES RELATED TO NOISE

The two key questions seek to determine whether the task does or does not call for verbal communications with co-workers or other people (for work purposes). In either case, both sections of the work sheet must be completed by answering simple questions that indirectly indicate noise levels:

- The noise bothers a little, but it is possible to talk to co-workers (or with the interviewer in the absence of co-workers).
- The noise is maddening, it is difficult to talk to co-workers (or with the interviewer in the absence of co-workers).
- The noise is very loud, and it is impossible to talk to co-workers (or with the interviewer in the absence of co-workers).

Depending on whether the task requires verbal communications with co-workers, the results will produce different scores, which will be depicted as different colored traffic lights representing this risk (Figure 4.7).

D	KEY-QUESTIONS FOR IDENTIFYING UV RADIATION BY OUTDOOR WORK OR WELDING WORK-RELATED PROBLEMS		
Exposure to UV radiation (welding) and/or sunlight UV radiations			
	Please, answer the following questions		
INDOOR WORK			
OCCASIONAL OUTDOOR WORK			
OUTDOOR WORK FOR A SIGNIFICANT PROPORTION OF THE YEAR (1/3) or WELDING AT LOW UV RADIATION RISK			
OUTDOOR WORK FOR MORE THAN HALF THE YEAR (2/3) or WELDING AT MEDIUM UV RADIATION RISK			
OUTDOOR WORK NEARLY ALL YEAR (3/3) or WELDING AT HIGHT UV RADIATION RISK			

FIGURE 4.6 Key questions for identifying issues related to exposure to ultraviolet (UV) radiation.

| E | KEY-QUESTIONS FOR IDENTIFYING HAZARDS RELATING TO NOISE |

Perceived noise level

Please, answer the following questions

The task calls for verbal communications with colleagues	
THE NOISE DOES NOT BOTHER	
THE NOISE BOTHERS A LITTLE, BUT IT IS POSSIBLE TO TALK TO COLLEAGUES	
THE NOISE IS MADDENING, IT IS DIFFICULT TO TALK TO COLLEAGUES	
THE NOISE IS VERY LOUD, IT IS IMPOSSIBLE TO TALK TO COLLEAGUES	

The task does not call for any verbal communications with colleagues	
THE NOISE DOES NOT BOTHER	
THE NOISE BOTHERS A LITTLE, BUT IT IS POSSIBLE TO TALK TO COLLEAGUES	
THE NOISE IS MADDENING, IT IS DIFFICULT TO TALK TO COLLEAGUES	
THE NOISE IS VERY LOUD, IT IS IMPOSSIBLE TO TALK TO COLLEAGUES	
NOTES	

FIGURE 4.7   Key questions for identifying issues related to noise.

4.6   KEY QUESTIONS FOR IDENTIFYING MICROCLIMATE-RELATED PROBLEMS

The first question asks whether the indoor and/or outdoor weather conditions are satisfactory all year round (Figure 4.8).

If the answer is NO, the next questions concern the microclimate inside the work place.

The key questions are very simple: Is it hot? Is it cold? Does this apply only in summer? Only in winter? All year?

There is also a question about whether the work is mainly outdoors (e.g. agriculture, construction) resulting in exposure to unfavorable weather conditions for part of the year (seasons too hot or too cold) or all year. If necessary, the type of unfavorable weather conditions can be described in the notes, especially with regard to work performed outdoors all year.

| F | KEY-QUESTIONS FOR IDENTIFYING MICROCLIMATE-RELATED PROBLEMS |

WORKING INDOORS WITH NO EXPOSURE TO THE WEATHER   Please, answer the following questions

COMFORTABLE ALL YEAR		
IT IS HOT:	ONLY IN SUMMER	
	ALL YEAR	
IT IS COLD:	ONLY IN WINTER	
	ALL YEAR	

WORKING OUTDOORS WITH EXPOSURE TO THE WEATHER

ONLY IN SUMMER	
ONLY IN WINTER	
ALL YEAR	
NOTES	

FIGURE 4.8   Key questions for identifying issues related to microclimate.

4.7 KEY QUESTIONS FOR IDENTIFYING PROBLEMS ARISING FROM THE USE OF EQUIPMENT/TOOLS

This section reports on the leading "intrinsic" issues relating to tools or equipment (heavy, noisy, require force, etc.); or which are problematic in relation to their use (technologically backward, require excessive attention, can cause injury, etc.). If present, an "X" will be placed in the box corresponding to the relevant problem (Figure 4.9).

4.8 KEY QUESTIONS FOR IDENTIFYING PROBLEMS RELATED TO EXPOSURE TO VIBRATIONS

A distinction is made between vibrations resulting from the use of tools (screwdrivers, grinders, cutters, pneumatic drills for at least 1/3 of the time) or from driving vehicles (whole-body vibrations for most of the time) (Figure 4.10).

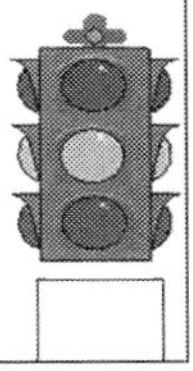

FIGURE 4.9 Key questions for identifying problems arising from the use of equipment/tools.

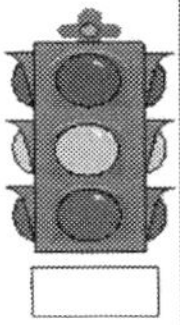

FIGURE 4.10 Key questions for identifying problems related to exposure to vibrations (hand-arm or whole body).

4.9 KEY QUESTIONS FOR IDENTIFYING PROBLEMS RELATED TO THE USE OF MACHINERY OR MACHINE PARTS

As for the section on tools and equipment, this section reports the most frequent "intrinsic" issues relating to machinery or parts of a machine, or which are problematic in relation to their use. If present, an "X" will be placed in the box corresponding to the relevant problem.

At times, it may be difficult to decide whether a tool is also a machine (e.g. a brush-cutter). Leaving aside the formal aspects, in such cases it will be necessary to choose whether to consider a tool as a machine or not, and work sheet (i) or (g) will be used accordingly. It is important to note that work sheets (i) and (g) cannot be used to describe the same equipment (Figure 4.11).

4.10 KEY ENTERS FOR IDENTIFYING PROBLEMS RELATED TO POLLUTANTS (CHEMICAL AGENTS, PARTICULATE, BIOLOGICAL AGENTS)

The key questions for this important section may seem excessively simple: they seek to determine if a potential pollutant is present and, if so, if it is present in large quantities. It should be emphasized that in addition to this work sheet, if a pollutant is reported, another work sheet must also be completed that provides preliminary information about the risk potential of such pollutants (see Chapter 6 on *quick assessments*) (Figure 4.12).

The same goes for the possible presence of biological agents (accidental or for deliberate use): the key enter is inserted in this section and then the special *quick assessment* work sheet (see Chapter 7) must be filled in accordingly.

It is vital to note that this questionnaire does not represent or replace the full Risk Assessment Document. The possible reporting of a hazard related to exposure to chemical agents (as for other hazardous situations) is a warning signal, which must necessarily be followed up with a thorough assessment based on the reference standards, and in the light of the technical and scientific evidence available at the time.

I KEY-QUESTIONS FOR IDENTIFYING PROBLEMS ARISING FROM THE USE OF MACHINERY	
	Please, answer the following questions
ADEQUATE AND KEPT IN GOOD CONDITION	
REQUIRES STRENGTH	
INVOLVES LIFTING HEAVY COMPONENTS	
NOISY	
NOT OPERATING PROPERLY	
NOT FIT FOR SPECIFIC USE AND/OR TECHNOLOGICALLY BACKWARD	
REQUIRES EXCESSIVE ATTENTION	
LIMITED SPACE AROUND MACHINERY	
MAY PRODUCE LESIONS (CUTS, SCRAPES, BLISTERS, BURNS, ETC.)	

FIGURE 4.11   Key questions for identifying problems related to the use of machinery or machine parts.

J	KEY-QUESTIONS FOR IDENTIFYING PROBLEMS ASSOCIATED WITH BIOLOGICAL OR OTHER POLLUTANTS		
			Please answer the following questions
NO BIOLOGICAL OR OTHER POLLUTANTS PRESENT			
DUST: specify type		PRESENT	
		SIGNIFICANT PRESENCE	
FUMES: specify type		PRESENT	
		SIGNIFICANT PRESENCE	
UNPLEASANT ODORS: describe		PRESENT	
		SIGNIFICANT PRESENCE	
CHEMICALS: specify type		PRESENT	
		SIGNIFICANT PRESENCE	
BIOLOGICAL POLLUTANTS		PRESENT	
		SIGNIFICANT PRESENCE	
NOTES			

FIGURE 4.12 Key enters for identifying problems related to pollutants (chemical agents, particulate, biological agents).

4.11 KEY ENTERS FOR IDENTIFYING ORGANIZATIONAL PROBLEMS AND WORK-RELATED STRESS

With regard to these aspects, which also include shift work, working hours and work pace, versus previous versions, it was decided not to provide specific key enters but to deal with them in a dedicated quick assessment sheet (Chapter 8).

This is specifically indicated here in Figure 4.13.

K	KEY-ENTERS FOR WORK ORGANIZATION AND STRESS
	To address these issues, go straight to work sheet "STRESS-ORG" Even if there is no suspicion of work-related STRESS, please fill in the sections on WORK ORGANIZATION (sections 1.2 and 1.3)

FIGURE 4.13 Advice for dealing with organizational issues (work-related stress, shift work, work pace, shift duration).

5 Second-Level Pre-mapping (*Quick Assessment*) for Studying Biomechanical Overload

Daniela Colombini and Enrico Occhipinti
Ergonomics of Posture and Movements
International Ergonomics School (EPM-IES)

CONTENTS

This chapter focusses on the *quick assessment* phase of various potential biomechanical overload conditions (from repetitive movements of the upper limbs to manual handling of loads (MHL) and awkward postures); a separate work sheet is used for each one.

With regard to the first two aspects (repetitive movements and MHL), the criteria set out in ISO/TR 12295 (ISO, 2014) have been followed, but the approach is aimed at determining priorities also for dealing with intermediate conditions that are neither "definitely acceptable" nor "definitely critical", according to same ISO Technical Report.

As already mentioned, since the ISO/TR does not provide any specific recommendations for conducting a *quick assessment* of working postures (for the trunk and lower limbs), the authors came up with an original re-interpretation of the criteria included in ISO 11226 (ISO, 2000) and EN 1005-4 (CEN, 2005), and the latest and most respected scientific literature on the subject. (Colombini and Occhipinti, 2017, 2019)

5.1 ANALYSIS OF THE UPPER LIMBS IN THE PRESENCE OF REPETITIVE MOVEMENTS

Once *key enters* have established that the work involves repetitive tasks, the relevant work sheet is filled in.

The first part of the work sheet refers to certain organizational aspects (Figure 5.1): shift duration, number and actual duration of breaks and duration of non-repetitive tasks. The purpose of this section is to determine how long the worker spends performing repetitive tasks during the shift; in other words, the *net duration of repetitive work*.

The second part (Figure 5.2) proposes a number of set scenarios which, when present simultaneously, allow the risk associated with repetitive work performed by the homogeneous group of workers to be defined as acceptable (*code green*).

B1-BIOMECHANICAL OVERLOAD DUE TO REPETITIVE MOVEMENTS

REPETITIVE TASK is present. DEFINITION: the task is organized in cycles, regardless of their duration or the task is characterized by similar gestures for over 50% of the time. The term "repetitive" does indicate the presence of risk. | YES

Summary of repetitive work net duration on a representative average day

TOTAL shift average duration (in minutes)	0	Total repetitive working time (in minutes)	0

DESCRIPTION OF NON-REPETITIVE TASKS, THEIR DURATION AND TIMING OF BREAKS - TOTAL DURATION

supply	0
cleaning	0
other	0
Total duration of non repetitive work per shift (in minutes)	0
Breaks (average) total duration per shift (in minutes): including meal break only if included in the shift	0
Number of breaks (including meal break) lasting\s at least 8 minutes	0

FIGURE 5.1 Quick risk assessment of upper limbs repetitive movements: organizational data.

ACCEPTABLE CONDITIONS

If all conditions are described and replies are all **"YES"**, the risk level is acceptable for repetitive work and it is not necessary to continue the risk evaluation.

NB: Please answer all questions by placing an "X" only in the blank spaces

			ACCEPTABLE	
Are one or both upper limbs used less than 50% of the total duration of the repetitive task(s)?	**No**		**Yes**	
Are both elbows held below shoulder level almost 90% of the total duration of the repetitive task(s)?	**No**		**Yes**	
Is moderate or no force required (perceived effort = max 3 or 4 on CR-10 Borg scale) by the operator for no more than 1 hour during the duration of the repetitive task(s) and are there no force peaks (perceived effort = 5 or more on CR-10 Borg scale)?	**No**		**Yes**	
Are there breaks (including meal break) lasting at least 8 min every 2 hours and is the repetitive task performed less than 8 hours a day?	**No**		**Yes**	

FIGURE 5.2 Quick risk assessment of upper limbs repetitive movements: pre-defined scenarios for determining acceptable risk (*code green*).

The third part (Figure 5.3) proposes additional pre-defined scenarios in which, if even only one of the replies is positive, it can be stated that the repetitive work performed by the homogeneous group of workers entails critical high-risk conditions (*critical, code purple*).

In short, the *quick assessment* work sheet for repetitive work will lead to the following three conclusions:

- The repetitive work is *acceptable in terms of risk* because the scenarios reported in the *code green* section have all been checked.
- The repetitive work is *definitely at risk* if even only one of the replies in the *critical code* section has been checked. In this case, remedial action must be urgently taken especially with regard to the critical aspects that have been checked. A risk assessment should also be conducted using the classic evaluation tools (Occupational Repetitive Action, OCRA checklist, or the even more precise OCRA Index) (ISO, 2007b; Colombini and Occhipinti, 2014, 2017).
- The repetitive work *could be at risk* because there are one or more significative replies in the scenarios listed in the *code green* section. A risk assessment must be performed using the classic evaluation tools (OCRA checklist or, for level four, the more precise OCRA Index); the situation is potentially a *code yellow* or *red* or also *purple*.

In actual fact, when conditions are neither acceptable nor critical, a simple scheme is recommended (Figure 5.4), which leads to a rough preliminary estimate of the OCRA checklist score range that might be expected from a more detailed analysis. As previously discussed in case of the *key enters*, the results of this *quick assessment* do not produce a score, but rather colors indicating the level of risk and priorities for the corrective actions.

CRITICAL CONDITIONS				
If at least one of the following conditions is present (**YES**), risk must be considered as CRITICAL and task redesign is URGENTLY REQUIRED. *NB. Please answer all the questions by placing an "X" only in the blank spaces*				
			CRITICAL	
Are technical actions performed with a single limb so fast that they cannot be counted by simple direct observation?	**No**		**Yes**	
Are one or both arms used to perform the task with elbow(s) at shoulder level for half or more than the total repetitive working time?	**No**		**Yes**	
Is a "pinch" grip (or any type of grasp using the finger tips) held for more than 80% of the repetitive working time?	**No**		**Yes**	
Is peak force applied (perceived effort = 5 or more on the CR-10 Borg scale) for 10% or more of the total repetitive working time?	**No**		**Yes**	
Is there only one break (including meal break) in a shift of 6-8 hours, or does the total repetitive working time exceed 8 hours in the shift?	**No**		**Yes**	

FIGURE 5.3 Quick risk assessment of upper limbs repetitive movements: pre-defined scenarios for determining the presence of high-risk conditions (*code critical, purple*).

Are there other risk factors to be considered when neither critical conditions nor acceptable conditions are present?				
Frequency				
Slow, medium or high frequency of technical actions performed with the dominant hand				
Slow (no more than 1 action every 2 seconds)	No		Yes	
Medium (no more than 1 action per second) or holding an object in the hands most	No		Yes	
High (more than 1 action per second): difficult to count actions	No		Yes	
Pace				
Is the pace mainly determined by the machine?	No		Yes	
Awkward postures				
Shoulder	Are the arms used with the elbow at shoulder level from one third to half of the total repetitive working time?	No		Yes
Hand	Is a "pinch" grip (or any kind of grasp using the finger tips) used from half to 80% of the repetitive working time?	No		Yes
Wrist	Are extreme wrist movements (flexion, extension or lateral deviations) required almost the whole time?	No		Yes
Elbow	Are extreme forearm movements (elbow flexion-extension or rotation) required almost the whole time?	No		Yes
Lack of variation				
Are the same actions and gestures repeated most of the time? Or is the cycle time very short (less than 8 sec.)?	No		Yes	
Use of force				
Is peak force (perceived effort = 5 or more on the CR-10 Borg scale) applied from 1% to 9 % of the time?	No		Yes	
Is moderate force (perceived effort = max 3 or 4 on CR-10 Borg scale) required by the operator?	No		Yes	
		Duration of MODERATE force	1/3 of time	

FIGURE 5.4   Quick risk assessment of upper limbs repetitive movements when conditions are neither acceptable nor critical.

In order to define the intervals of these color scales, potential OCRA checklist values have been calculated for each scenario, so that when the work sheets are completed, the system generates a kind of *pre-index* (not visible to the compiler) in which:

- *green* (less than 7.5) means acceptable risk.
- *yellow* (7.5–11) means potential risk, to be assessed but not as a high priority.
- *red* (11.1–22.5) means risk probably present, and situation to be assessed.
- *purple* (more than 22.5) means risk definitely present and assessment urgently required.

The maximum score for this concealed *pre-index* is 25, and the percentage of biomechanical load is calculated with respect to this value: this ratio will later be used to briefly define the extent to which the upper limbs are engaged with respect to other risk factors.

Once compiled, a summary of the assessment appears at the bottom of the work sheet in the ERGOCHECK program with an indication of the relevant action priorities (Figure 5.5).

BIOMECHANICAL OVERLOAD OF UPPER LIMBS IN REPETITIVE TASKS	
SUMMARY OF PRE-ASSESSMENT AND INTERVENTION PRIORITIES	

FIGURE 5.5 Summary of *quick assessment* for repetitive movements.

5.2 *QUICK ASSESSMENT* OF MANUAL LOAD LIFTING

Once the key enter has determined that the work entails manual load lifting, the specific *quick assessment* work sheet needs to be completed.

The first part of the work sheet requires specific questions to be asked (about certain characteristics of the environment, the objects lifted or carried and the work organization) that could represent additional risk factors in load lifting tasks (Figure 5.6) and that must be considered in the assessment, in accordance with Annex I to EU Directive 269/90/EEC.

The second part (Figure 5.7) suggests predefined scenarios: if even one of the answers is positive, the lifting work involves critical conditions with high-risk exposure (*code critical, purple*).

These are the scenarios for which the revised NIOSH lifting equation (Waters et al., 1993) proposes "Ø" as the multiplier for calculating the recommended weight (in practice, in these scenarios the recommended weight is equal to Ø kg, i.e. manual lifting should be avoided). Such situations include: distance from the body greater than 63 cm, height of the hands at the origin and the destination of the lift greater than 175 cm, etc.

A condition is also considered to be critical when a single employee has to manually lift loads exceeding the maximum lifting limits suggested, by gender and age, by the technical standards ISO 11228-1 and EN1005-2 (ISO, 2003; CEN, 2003) and Annex A of ISO/TR 12295 (ISO, 2014).

The third section (Figure 5.8) proposes predefined scenarios which, if all are present (i.e. positive answers) mean that the lifting work performed by the homogeneous group is associated with an acceptable exposure level (*code green*).

Additional ORGANIZATIONAL AND ENVIROMENTAL risk factors		
Is the working environment unfavorable for manual lifting and carrying?		
Presence of extreme (low or high) temperatures	No	Yes
Presence of slippery, uneven, unstable floors	No	Yes
Presence of insufficient space for lifting and carrying	No	Yes
Are objects unfavorable for manual lifting and carrying?		
The size of object reduces the operator's view and hinders movement	No	Yes
The centre of gravity of the load is not stable (for example: liquids, items moving around inside the object)	No	Yes
The object's shape/configuration features sharp edges, surfaces or protrusions	No	Yes
The contact surfaces are too cold or too hot	No	Yes
Does the task with manual lifting or carrying last more than 8 hours a day?	No	Yes

FIGURE 5.6 Quick risk assessment of manual lifting and carrying: preliminary evaluation of certain unfavorable characteristics of the organization, environment and objects handled.

CRITICAL CONDITIONS if only one of aforementioned conditions is present (YES), the risk is to be considered as high and the task must be immediately re-designed.					
Task lay-out and frequency					
VERTICAL LOCATION	The hand location at the beginning/end of the lift is higher than 175 cm or lower than 0 cm	No		Yes	
VERTICAL DISPLACEMENT	The vertical distance between the origin and the destination of the lifted object is more than 175cm	No		Yes	
HORIZONTAL DISTANCE	The horizontal distance between the body and load is greater than full arm reach	No		Yes	
ASYMMETRY	Extreme body twisting without moving the feet	No		Yes	
FREQUENCY	equal to or higher than 15 times/minute for SHORT DURATION (MAX 60 min)	No		Yes	
	equal to or higher than 12 times/minute for MEDIUM DURATION (MAX 120 min)	No		Yes	
	equal to or higher than 8 times/minute for LONG DURATION (OVER 120 min)	No		Yes	
Presence of loads exceeding the following limits					
men (18-45 years)		No		Yes	
women (18-45 years)		No		Yes	
men (<18 or >45 years)		No		Yes	
women (<18 or >45 years)		No		Yes	

FIGURE 5.7 Quick risk assessment of manual lifting: pre-defined scenarios for determining the presence of high risk: (*critical code, purple*).

ACCEPTABLE CONDITIONS If there are NO LOADS >10KG and all underreported conditions are fulfilled and replies are all **YES** (using both hands in lifting) for every weight category present (<10KG), the risk level is acceptable for manual lifting loads. **However, additional factors must also be checked (see above).** NB. Please answer all questions by placing an "X" only in the blank spaces					
Are there loads weighing between 3 and 5 KG?		No		Yes	
3 to 5 KG loads	Asymmetry (e.g. body rotation, trunk twisting) is absent	No		Yes	
	Load is maintained close to the body	No		Yes	
	Load vertical displacement is between hips and shoulders	No		Yes	
	Maximum frequency: less than 5 lifts per minute	No		Yes	
Are there loads weighing between 5 and 10 KG?		No		Yes	
5 to 10 KG loads	Asymmetry (e.g. body rotation, trunk twisting) is absent	KG		Yes	
	Load is maintained close to the body	No		Yes	
	Load vertical displacement is between hips and shoulders	No		Yes	
	Maximum frequency: less than 5 lifts per minute	No		Yes	
Are loads weighing more than 10 KG lifted?		No		Yes	

FIGURE 5.8 Quick risk assessment of manual lifting risk: pre-defined scenarios for determining the presence of acceptable risk: (*code green*).

These scenarios involve manual lifting of loads weighing up to 10 kg with almost "ideal" lifting frequencies and workplace structures.

However, in this case, no objects must weigh more than 10 kg and this must be indicated by answering "YES" to the question in Figure 5.8: "Are there loads weighing more than 10 kg?"

In short, the *quick assessment* work sheet for analyzing tasks that involve manual load lifting will, as in the case of repetitive movements, lead to one of the following three conclusions:

- The manual lifting work is at *acceptable risk* because all the scenarios listed in the *green code* section are checked.
- Manual load lifting work *could be at risk* because there are one or more positive replies in the scenarios listed in the *code green* section; a risk assessment should be conducted using the classic evaluation tools (revised NIOSH lifting equation).
- The manual load lifting work is *definitely at risk* if even only one of the replies in scenarios for the *critical code* section is positive. Upgrades or remedial action must be undertaken urgently with regard to the conditions defined as critical, to be followed by a risk assessment using one of the classic evaluation tools (revised NIOSH lifting equation).

In order to complete the analysis of lifting tasks through the use of *green codes* and *critical codes*, other scenarios have been added to more comprehensively describe the handling of objects of different weights (Figure 5.9). As in the case of repetitive movements, with this additional information, it will be possible to more accurately determine the color scale score and degree of biomechanical engagement of the spine with respect to the pre-defined maximum scores.

As previously seen for the *key enters*, the results of this *quick assessment* do not generate a visible score, but rather color scales indicating the level of risk and priorities for the corrective action plan.

If even only one of the scenarios on the *critical code* list is positive, the color scale moves towards *purple*. Having pre-defined the *maximum value* (taking into account problems relating to the environment, load characteristics, workplace layout and organizational set-up), the degree of biomechanical effort is calculated with respect to this maximum threshold. As for all causes of risk, this ratio is used to briefly define the degree of involvement of the spine in manual load lifting tasks.

Characteristics and frequency of certain loads (more than 10 KG)				
Please, mark the weight category present, or check the previous question				
Are there loads weighing between 10 and 15 KG?			No	Yes
10.5 to 15 KG loads	Asymmetry (e.g. body rotation, trunk twisting) is absent		No	Yes
	Load is maintained close to the body		No	Yes
	Load vertical displacement is between hips and shoulders		No	Yes
	Maximum frequency: less than 1 lift every 5 minutes		No	Yes
Are there loads weighted more than 15 kg up to 25 kg?			No	Yes
15.51 to 25 KG loads	Asymmetry (e.g. body rotation, trunk twisting) is absent		No	Yes
	Load is maintained close to the body		No	Yes
	Load vertical displacement is between hips and shoulders		No	Yes
	Maximum frequency: less than 1 lift every 5 minutes		No	Yes

FIGURE 5.9 Quick risk assessment of manual lifting: pre-defined scenarios for completing the description of lifting conditions.

5.3 *QUICK ASSESSMENT* OF MANUAL LOAD CARRYING TASKS

For the *quick assessment*, the calculation of the *cumulative mass* (as per ISO 11228-1) (ISO, 2003) has been used, i.e. the total weight of all the loads carried per shift, per hour or per minute. The *cumulative mass carried* is compared with the *tolerable cumulative mass carried for 8 hours, 1 hour, and 1 minute*: a critical situation arises (*critical code, purple*) if the load exceeds the tolerated weight. The *tolerated cumulative mass* varies according to the distance and the duration scenario; for example, the threshold is 10,000 kg for 8 hours but drops to 6,000 kg for loads carried over a distance of more than 10 m.

Nonetheless the condition is considered *critical* when objects are carried that individually weigh more than the limits, by gender and age, indicated for lifting; in fact, as suggested by ISO 11228-1 in most cases the carrying task is preceded by a lifting action and concludes with a depositing action.

To estimate the *cumulative mass carried*, it is necessary to specify the time (in minutes) dedicated to carrying (or lifting+carrying), the number of objects carried in the shift, their weight (at least broken down by categories) and the "modal" carrying distance covered. The calculation is made automatically and the results (kg of cumulated mass carried) will be compared with the maximum acceptable results for 8-hour, 1-hour, and 1-minute scenarios, as per the specific table in ISO 11228-1. The percentage of the *cumulative mass carried* in relation to the cumulative mass tolerated is calculated as a "hidden" value.

It should also be noted that, since ISO 11228-1 is under revision and the *quick assessment* criteria for carrying are likely to be amended, the section on *quick assessments* for carrying tasks will be updated as soon as the new version of the ISO standard is adopted (Figure 5.10).

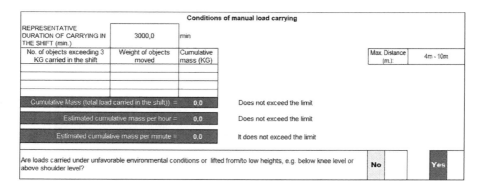

FIGURE 5.10 Quick risk assessment of manual carrying: estimation of *cumulative mass carried* in 8-hour, 1-hour and 1-minute scenarios; comparison with relative acceptability limits.

5.4 *QUICK ASSESSMENT* OF MANUAL PUSHING AND/OR PULLING

Figure 5.11 lists the conditions to be examined first of all to define the manual pushing or pulling of trolleys or trans-pallets as acceptable. These conditions could in fact represent additional risk factors in load handling work and must be taken into due consideration in the evaluation, as required by Annex I to EU Directive 269/90/EEC.

Figure 5.12 describes the conditions for assessing manual pushing and pulling tasks as acceptable. The conditions in Figure 5.12 must all be met (together with the previous ones in Figure 5.11) to conclude that the pushing and/or pulling work is acceptable (*code green*).

If even just one of the conditions shown in Figure 5.13 is present, manual pushing or pushing will be defined as critical, regardless of whether or not the more complex assessment methods included in ISO 11228-2 (ISO, 2007a) and ISO/TR 12295-Annex B (ISO, 2014) are used.

With regard to the *quick assessment* of manual pushing and pulling, it should be noted that the Borg scale (CR-10 version) is used for estimating the important parameter of the intensity of perceived effort (or force) (Borg, 1998).

IS THERE WHOLE-BODY PUSHING OR PULLING OF LOADS?			
NB: IF PRESENT, SPECIFY THE BORG SCALE VALUE IN THE WHITE BOX BELOW			
Perceived effort (obtained by interviewing workers using the CR-10 Borg scale):		**3,0 - moderate**	
Additional organizational and enviromental risk factors to be considered			
Is the working environment unfavourable for pushing or pulling?			
Are floors slippery, unstable, uneven, upward or downward sloping or cracked/broken?	No		Yes
Are there restricted or obstructed paths?	No		Yes
Is the temperature of the working area high?	No		Yes
Are objects unfavorable for pushing or pulling?			
Does the object (or trolley, pallet, etc.) limit the view of the operator or hinder movement?	No		Yes
Is the object unstable?	No		Yes
Does the object (or trolley, pallet, etc.) have hazardous features, sharp surfaces, projections etc. that could injure the operator?	No		Yes
Are the wheels or casters worn, broken or not properly maintained?	No		Yes
Are the wheels or casters unsuitable for the working conditions?	No		Yes

FIGURE 5.11 Quick risk assessment of manual pushing and pulling: preliminary evaluation of certain unfavorable characteristics of the environment and objects pushed or pulled.

ACCEPTABLE CONDITIONS			
If all conditions are met and replies are all YES, the risk level is acceptable for pushing-pulling tasks. However, **additional factors must also be checked (see above). NB. Please answer all questions by placing an "X" only in the blank spaces**			
Does the perceived effort (obtained by interviewing workers using the CR-10 Borg scale) show the presence during pushing-pulling task(s) of up to SLIGHT exertion (perceived effort - score 2 or less in Borg CR-10 scale)?	No		Yes
Is the manual pushing and pulling work performed for up to 8 hours a day?	No		Yes
Is pushing-pulling force applied to the object between hip and mid-chest height?	No		Yes
Is the pushing-pulling work performed with an upright trunk (not twisted or bent)?	No		Yes
Are hands held within shoulder width and in front of the body?	No		Yes

FIGURE 5.12 Quick risk assessment of manual pushing and pulling: pre-defined scenarios for determining the presence of acceptable risk: (*code green*).

CRITICAL CONDITIONS				
if even only one of these conditions is present (YES), the risk is to be considered as high and the task must be				
NB: Please answer all questions by placing an "X" only in the blank spaces				
Does the perceived effort using the CR-10 Borg scale (obtained by interviewing the workers) show the presence of high peaks of force (perceived effort, with a score of 8 or more on the Borg CR-10 scale)?	No		Yes	
Is the pushing-pulling work performed with the trunk significantly bent or twisted?	No		Yes	
Is the pushing-pulling work performed in a jerky or uncontrolled manner?	No		Yes	
Are hands held either wider than shoulder width or not in front of the body?	No		Yes	
Hands are held higher than 150 cm or lower than 60 cm.	No		Yes	
Together with the pushing-pulling work is there also use of vertical force ("partial lifting")?	No		Yes	
Does the task(s) with manual pushing and pulling lasts more than 8 hours a day?	No		Yes	

FIGURE 5.13 Quick risk assessment of manual pushing and pulling: pre-defined scenarios for determining the presence of high risk: (*critical code, purple*).

When the Borg scale level is equal to or less than 2 (light effort/force), the condition may be acceptable while, if the level is equal to or greater than 8, the condition is definitely critical.

It is useful to collect the workers' perceptions (better still measured using the Borg CR-10 scale) for pushing and pulling activities. This also makes it possible to gauge intermediate conditions (Borg scale between 3 and 7) that are definitely not acceptable but not yet definitely critical as estimated on the basis of the percentage of force used.

In many cases, this approach can overcome, at least initially and through a participatory but facilitated approach, the issue of conducting measurements using a dynamometer during pushing or pulling tasks.

Lastly, it should be noted that a summary of the assessment appears at the bottom of the work sheet on MHL, for each completed section (lifting, carrying, pulling/pushing, and additional factors for lifting/carrying and pushing/pulling), indicating the relevant action priorities (Figure 5.14). In this section, the summary for additional

Summary of quick assessment for manual load handling	
BIOMECHANICAL OVERLOAD FOR MANUAL LIFTING	
SUMMARY OF PRE-ASSESSMENT AND INTERVENTION PRIORITIES	
BIOMECHANICAL OVERLOAD FOR MANUAL CARRYING	
SUMMARY OF PRE-ASSESSMENT AND INTERVENTION PRIORITIES	
Summary of enviromental additional factors important for MMH	
BIOMECHANICAL OVERLOAD FOR PUSHING and PULLING	
SUMMARY OF PRE-ASSESSMENT AND INTERVENTION PRIORITIES	
Summary of additional enviromental factors THAT ARE SIGNIFICANT for PUSHING and PULLING	

FIGURE 5.14 Summary of *quick assessment* for manual load handling.

factors is separate from the assessment proper. Conversely, as will be seen later, in the final section indicating the priorities of all risk factors, the priority for lifting/carrying and pushing/pulling, respectively, is determined also on the basis of an integration of additional factors and purely biomechanical aspects.

5.5 *QUICK ASSESSMENT* OF WORKING POSTURES

The *quick assessment* technique is used in the relative work sheet to evaluate postures and movements of the trunk and lower limbs. Postures and movements of the upper limbs are in fact evaluated in the previous work sheet for repetitive movements. Postures of the neck (cervical spine) are not assessed.

For each of the two segments analyzed here (trunk and lower limbs), there are specific figures illustrating more or less acceptable postures: the interviewer must indicate if a certain posture is present and estimate the percentage of time spent in that position in relation to the overall working time. For each segment, the sum of the percentages must add up to 100%

In the case of the trunk (Figure 5.15), an initial distinction must be made between standing and seated postures and the fraction of time spent in each position shown must be indicated. Since some work may be performed standing and some sitting, the percentages should be broken down between the relevant postures (with the sum total adding up to 100%).

The same goes for postures and movements of the lower limbs. Also in this case (Figure 5.16), the fractions of time (percentages) must be reported for the lower limbs with regard to standing and sitting positions, respectively.

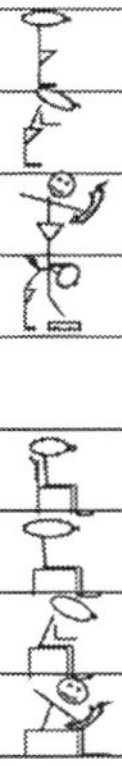

Trunk posture		
Standing or squatting (not seated)		% time
Nearly always upright		
Frequent moderate bending		
Frequent twisting		
Frequent deep bending		
Seated		
Leaning on the back rest		
Upright without backrest		
Mostly bending forward		
Frequent twisting of trunk		
Note:	described time of trunk posture:	0%

FIGURE 5.15 *Quick assessment* of postures and movements of the trunk.

Lower limb postures	
Standing or squatting (not seated)	% time
Standing and able to walk around	
Standing in a fixed posture	
Kneeling or crouching	
Sitting	% time
Leg room sufficient	
Leg room insufficient or very limited	
Leg room non-existent	
Note:	Described time of lower limbs posture 0%

FIGURE 5.16 *Quick assessment* of postures and movements of the lower limbs.

The final indication refers to the possible use and operation of pedals with one or both lower limbs (Figure 5.17). This information must be entered with the percentage of time spent not pressing and/or pressing pedals, respectively. Again, the fractions of time must add up to 100%.

At the bottom of the work sheet, there is a specific section (Figure 5.18) showing a summary of the evaluation of trunk and lower limb postures with an indication of the level of priority and consequent corrective actions.

Use of lower limbs	
	% time
No pedals used	
Lower limbs used to press pedals	
Note:	Duration of lower limb use 0%

FIGURE 5.17 *Quick assessment* of the use of pedals with the lower limbs.

BIOMECHANICAL OVERLOAD FROM AWKWARD POSTURES - TRUNK AND LOWER LIMBS	
SUMMARY OF PRE-ASSESSMENT AND INTERVENTION PRIORITIES	

FIGURE 5.18 Summary of the *quick assessment* of postures of the trunk and lower limbs.

6 Second-Level Pre-mapping (Quick Assessment) for the Preliminary Study of Exposure to Chemical Agents and Particulate

Daniela Colombini and Enrico Occhipinti
Ergonomics of Posture and Movements
International Ergonomics School (EPM-IES)

This chapter focusses on the risk of exposure in particular to chemical agents (substances or mixtures) as well as to particulate (dust and fumes).

Several approaches can be found in the literature and on the websites of numerous international agencies for the evaluation and simple management of exposure to chemicals; they generally go by the name of Control Banding.

According to the International Labour Organization (ILO), Control Banding is a complementary approach to protecting worker health (from chemical agents) by focussing resources on exposure management. Since it is not possible to assign a specific occupational exposure limit to every chemical in use, a chemical is assigned to a "band" for preventive measures, based on its hazard classification (according to international criteria), the amount of chemical in use and its volatility. The outcome is a recommended control and prevention strategy (ILO, 2018).

Control Banding was developed so that users can quickly determine appropriate measures for the protection of workers (e.g. replacement with less dangerous agents, modification of work practices and technological measures, selection and use of appropriate personal protective equipment), based on available information on the health risks posed by the agents, potential exposure and methods for exposure control. The procedures and schemes are mainly intended to be used by small- and medium-sized enterprises as a screening tool in the exposure assessment process.

Besides the aforementioned website of the ILO, which also operates in close synergy with the WHO on "Chemical Control Banding" (ILO, 2018), also worth mentioning is the website of the UK Health and Safety Executive (HSE), which adopts a more practical approach to the "Control of Substances Hazardous to Health

(COSHH)" (HSE, 2018) or the website of the International Occupational Hygiene Association (IOHA) that also deals with the same subject (IOHA, 2018).

These websites will provide interested readers with theoretical and practical information concerning the procedures for the simple assessment and management of "chemical risk".

Here, for the purposes of preliminary risk mapping, while endorsing and adopting the general rationale underpinning Control Banding, it was decided to take a less analytical approach towards analyzing chemical agents and particulates. This essentially means referring to general information on the hazardousness of substances (mainly from labeling), mode of use and quantities, in order to determine priorities for subsequent evaluations, which can then be performed using the actual Control Banding techniques (when appropriate and sufficient) or more detailed instrumental occupational toxicology measurements.

The pre-mapping work sheet (Figure 6.1) provides a list of possible chemicals and particulates, broken down into macro-categories, each of which may pose a health or accident risk. These are classified and grouped by means of *pictograms* and described by *H-phrases* (hazard statements) in accordance with *Regulation (EC) No. 1272/2008 of the European Parliament and Council of 16 December 2008,* published in the *Official Journal of the European Union* on 31 December 2008, on the classification, labeling and packaging of substances and mixtures.

	HEALTH RISKS FROM ACUTE EXPOSURE					HEALTH RISKS FROM CHRONIC EXPOSURE					SAFETY RISKS					
	EXTREMELY HIGH	HIGH	MEDIUM	LOW	SENSITIZATION RISK	EXTREMELY HIGH	HIGH	MEDIUM	LOW	SENSITIZATION RISK	EXTREMELY HIGH			HIGH	MEDIUM	LOW
	VERY TOXIC	TOXIC / CORROSIVE	HARMFUL	IRRITATING	SENSITIZING	CARCINOGENIC; MUTAGENIC; REPRODUCTIVE CYCLE RISK; TERATOGENIC	CARCINOGENIC; MUTAGENIC; REPRODUCTIVE RISK; TERATOGENIC; TOXIC	TOXIC	IRRITATING	SENSITIZING	EXPLOSION / EXTREMELY FLAMMABLE / COMBUSTIBLE			EASILY FLAMMABLE / EXPLOSIVE	FLAMMABLE	HIGH FLASH POINT (UE > 70°)
	H300 H310 H330	H301 H311 H331 / H314 H318	H302 H312 H332	H315 H319 H335	H317 H334	H340 H350 H360	H341 H361 H361 H370 H372	H371 H373	H315 H319 H335 OR WITHOUT "H" LABEL	H317 H334	H200 H201 H202 H203 H240 H241 / H220 H222 H224 H241 H222 H251 H252 / H260			H225 H228 / H204	H221 H226 (IN CERTAIN CONDITIONS)	NO LABEL
ACIDS																
BASES																
FUELS																
ORGANIC COMPOUNDS																
DUST																
GAS FUMES																
PLASTICS																
METALLOIDS AND METALS																
OXIDANTS																
PESTICIDES																
SOLVENTS																

FIGURE 6.1 Descriptive diagram of potential pollutants: identification of risk characteristics.

H-phrases may cover both *physical hazards* (e.g. H226 – Flammable liquid and vapors) and *health hazards* (e.g. H350 – May cause cancer and H335 – May irritate the respiratory tract).

While the health risks (both acute and chronic) are of greater interest here, the potential risk of accident (fire and explosion) associated with the substance in use is also reported in the work sheet.

The use of this part of the work sheet in Figure 6.1 is, for chemical compounds, fairly simple: it is a matter of reading the label of the product in use (or its technical

	BRIEF DESCRIPTION OF THE MANUFACTURING PROCESS IN ORDER TO CHARACTERIZE WORKER EXPOSURE					
	TYPE OF EXPOSURE			FREQUENCY OF EXPOSURE		
	CLOSED CYCLE / COMPLETE	CONTROLLED CYCLE / INHALATION/SEPARATION??	OPEN CYCLE / DIRECT CONTACT AND HANDLING	OCCASIONAL (not every day)	LOW BUT DAILY	HIGH AND DAILY
ACIDS						
BASES						
FUELS						
ORGANIC COMPOUNDS						
DUSTS						
GAS FUMES						
PLASTICS						
METALLOIDS AND METALS						
ODIXANTS						
PESTICIDES						
SOLVENTS						

FIGURE 6.2 Descriptive diagram of potential pollutants: semi-quantitative description of exposure.

data sheet) and placing an "X" in the column with the *pictogram* and the corresponding *H-phrase*.

In the case of particulates (fumes and dust), the approach will be the same, even if there are no technical data sheets.

Once the presence of the chemical has been recognized and classified (qualitative data), the description is completed with the relevant quantitative data (Figure 6.2). The exposure may be described as: *closed-cycle, controlled-cycle or involve direct handling*. The frequency of exposure will be reported as *sporadic, short but daily* or *high and daily*.

With regard to the "concealed scores", descriptive scores are attributed from the highest to the lowest risk products. The scores are also adjusted for the quantitative degree of exposure.

At the bottom of the page, there is a summary of the pre-assessment, which indicates the level of priority for conducting a more in-depth evaluation.

7 Second-Level Pre-mapping (Quick Assessment) for the Preliminary Study of Exposure to Biological Agents

Ugo Caselli
INAIL

CONTENTS

7.1 OBJECTIVES AND LIMITS

Managing the risk of exposure to biological agents poses a number of significant problems, especially in the risk assessment phase, since standardized methods cannot be used primarily due to the unavailability of reference standards and limits. In fact, the issue is at best poorly understood in most sectors, with the exception of health care, including the livestock and waste collection and disposal sectors, where it deserves to be dealt with in depth. Hence the need for easy-to-use preliminary tools that can be used even by non-experts in the field of biological risk, enabling employers and prevention and protection services to determine if the workplace or individual task may be characterized as critical due to the presence of biological agents.

These considerations were the rationale that led to the creation of the pre-mapping work sheet for biological agents presented and illustrated in this chapter, the aim being to develop an initial easy-to-use screening tool for use by anyone involved in the management of workplace health and safety. This tool provides guidance as whether or not to conduct a comprehensive assessment of risk due to biological agents; it does not pretend to replace the assessment itself, but rather provides a preliminary introduction to the problem. The aim is to help even non-specialists identify potential criticalities. The work sheet provides an indication of potential exposure to biological agents in the form of a bar graph and compares the results with other types of risks.

7.2 PRE-MAPPING WORK SHEET

Pre-mapping, which can be found in point (j) of the general framework (Chapter 4, Figure 4.12), draws a distinction between the deliberate use of biological agents and the potential/occasional presence of a biological agent in the working environment/ production facility. If even one of the two cases is present, then a more in-depth analysis is required using the "BIOLOGICAL" work sheet.

There are three parts in the "BIOLOGICAL" work sheet:

- The first section (A) focusses on the deliberate use of biological agents belonging to groups 1, 2, 3 and 4 in the workplace.
- The second section (B) aims to detect potential criticalities in the workplace (description of scenarios and activities that could present potential risks), both in relation to the deliberate use of biological agents or their potential or occasional presence.
- The third section (C) should be used if the workers develop diseases or disorders due to exposure to biological agents.

Of course, when use of biological agents is intentional or deliberate, all 3 sections (A, B, C) need to be filled in, while if there may be potential or incidental use of such agents, only sections B and C need completing (not section A). Once completed, this work sheet generates a descriptive score: the higher the score, the more critical the situation for the workplace under examination.

7.2.1 SECTION A: DELIBERATE USE OF BIOLOGICAL AGENTS

If a workplace uses biological agents intentionally or deliberately, Section A first identifies the group to which the agents belong (group 1, 2, 3 or 4, depending on how hazardous they are) in accordance with Italian and European Legislation (Figure 7.1), and then quantifies the frequency of exposure. Frequency may be:

- Sporadic (once or twice a month or even less);
- Rare (no more than once or twice a week);
- Frequent (weekly but not daily);
- Very frequent (daily).

The score increases with the frequency of exposure, and the work sheet reflects the rating using colors (the traffic-light system).

BIOLOGICAL POLLUTANTS DELIBERATELY USED IN THE MANUFACTURING PROCESS (bacteria and similar organisms, parasites, fungi)	SPORADIC (1-2 times a month or less)	RARE (no more than 1-2 times a week)	FREQUENT (exposure weekly, but not daily)	VERY FREQUENT (exposure daily)
GROUP 1 BIOLOGICAL POLLUTANTS Generally unlikely to cause human disease AS PER ANNEX XLVI OF ITALIAN LEG. DECREE Nr. 81/08: (Saccharomyces cerevisiae, Streptococcus thermophylus, Lactobacillus casei, Staphylococcus xylosus, etc.)				
GROUP 2 BIOLOGICAL POLLUTANTS. May cause human disease and constitute a risk for workers; unlikely to spread to the community; effective prophylaxis or treatment generally available; AS PER ANNEX XLVI OF ITALIAN LEG. DECREE Nr. 81/08 (Campylobacter spp. Clostridium spp. Corynebacterium spp. Enterobacter spp. Klebsiella spp. Legionella spp. Salmonella paratyphi, Staphylococcus aureus, Streptococcus spp. Treponema spp. Cytomegalovirus, Measles virus, Mumps virus, duodenal Ancylostoma, Toxoplasma gondii, Candida albicans, etc.)				
GROUP 3 BIOLOGICAL POLLUTANTS. May cause severe human disease and constitute a serious risk for workers; may spread to the community; but effective prophylaxis or treatment generally available; AS PER ANNEX XLVI OF ITALIAN LEG. DECREE Nr. 81/08 (Bacillus anthracis, Brucella melitensis, Mycobacterium tuberculosis, Rickettsia rickettsii, Salmonella typhi, Yersinia pestis, Dengue virus, Nile virus, Yellow Fever virus, AIDS virus, Plasmodium falciparum, Taenia solium, etc.)				
GROUP 4 BIOLOGICAL POLLUTANTS. May cause severe human disease and constitute a serious risk for workers; at high risk of spreading to the community; no effective prophylaxis or treatment generally available; AS PER ANNEX XLVI OF ITALIAN LEG. DECREE Nr. 81/08 (Ebola virus, Lassa virus, Marburg virus, etc.)				

FIGURE 7.1 Section A: deliberate use of biological agents (Italian Legislative Decree no. 81/08).

7.2.2   SECTION B: DESCRIPTION OF SCENARIOS AND TASKS THAT COULD POSE POTENTIAL RISK (CRITICALITIES)

If biological agents are potentially or incidentally present, but also deliberately used in the workplace, it is necessary to identify one or more of the critical situations listed in section B. Each case is associated with a score, which increases in relation to both the level of risk involved and the frequency of exposure; the score is also rated using colors (traffic lights). If several critical situations are present, the final score will be the highest of all those indicated in the work sheet. The criticalities shown in Section B (Figure 7.2) refer both to specific work phases and to situations and peculiarities of the workplace in general, such as indoor plant and equipment, in outdoor environments and contact with wild animals.

7.2.3   SECTION C: TYPE AND NUMBER OF DISEASES AND DISORDERS DUE TO BIOLOGICAL AGENTS IN THE HOMOGENEOUS GROUP OF WORKERS

Section C should only be completed if the workers report diseases or disorders due to biological agents. The presence of such pathologies must be described qualitatively and quantitatively in relation to the homogeneous group (Figure 7.3).

7.3   FINAL SCORE AND CONCLUSIONS

The final score, also highlighted using colors (traffic lights present in the software), will indicate one of the following conditions:

- No further risk assessment is necessary (code green in the software);
- A further assessment of biological risk is advisable (code yellow in the software);
- Definite risk sources are present; therefore, a further risk assessment is necessary (code red in the software);
- High-priority critical conditions are present (code purple in the software).

The pre-mapping work sheet for biological agents represents an innovative and flexible tool that can be applied quickly and easily to take a sufficiently representative snapshot of the possible presence of criticalities in the workplace. This allows staff in charge of workplace health and safety, especially those without specific expertise in dealing with biological hazards, to verify the need for a more in-depth evaluation on the basis of the results obtained, so as to then implement the most appropriate prevention and protection measures.

The summary work sheet (ERGOCHECK final results) compares the outcome of this risk factor with that of other types of risk (depicted with bar graphs going from 0% to 100%) (see Chapter 9).

BIOLOGICAL POLLUTANTS POTENTIALLY PRESENT - CRITICALITIES (TO BE COMPLETED WHETHER OR NOT BIOLOGICAL POLLUTANTS ARE DELIBERATELY USED IN THE MANUFACTURING PROCESS)	SPORADIC (1-2 times a month or less)	RARE (no more than 1-2 times a week)	FREQUENT (exposure weekly, but not daily)	VERY FREQUENT (exposure daily)
Presence of centralized air conditioning system with air conditioning unit (AIR TREATMENT UNIT)				
Activities involving water nebulization (spas and wellness centers, showers, etc.)				
Activities involving contact with animals, feces and bio-aerosols deriving from same (farms, veterinary and grooming services, pest control, park rangers, etc.)				
Activities involving contact with products/substances derived from animals (farms, food industries, slaughterhouses, tanneries, dairies, kitchens, etc.)				
Activities involving contact with products/substances derived from plants (agriculture, food industries, paper mills, cosmetics, feed mills, wine cellars, oil presses, carpentry shops, kitchens etc.)				
Outdoor activities with potential risk of bites by insects, snakes, etc. (e.g. agriculture)				
Activities involving potential exposure to blood or other biological fluids (health care, child care, research and analytical laboratories, beauty salons, tattoo parlors)				
Activities involving the collection, management, treatment, recycling and/or disposal of solid or liquid urban/industrial waste and production of organic fertilizers				
Cleaning and disinfection activities (premises, equipment, materials, etc.) and/or laundering				
Activities involving the use of mineral oils (engineering, etc.)				
Construction activities, animal-free agriculture, involving contact with soil and/or plant- and animal-derived substances				
Plant maintenance activities (HVAC, etc.)				
Personal care services (kindergartens, nursing homes, barbershops and hairdressers, etc.)				
Activities involving the use of animal and plant metabolites (proteins, enzymes, etc.)				
Wholesalers / retailers excluding plant and animal derived products				
Activities in crowded environments such as schools, gyms etc. (lice, mite allergies ...)				
Transport and storage activities (excluding products of plant and animal origin)				
Manufacturing activities: textile, chemical, pharmaceutical, rubber and plastic industries, hydrocarbon refining or other on signaling.				

FIGURE 7.2 Section B: critical areas (description of scenarios and work activities that might present potential risks).

PRESENCE OF DISEASES IN THE HOMOGENEOUS GROUP CAUSED BY EXPOSURE TO BIOLOGICAL AGENTS: describe the type and number of diseases/disorders and tick the box below.

FIGURE 7.3 Section C: type and number of diseases and disorders due to biological agents in the homogeneous group.

8 Second-Level Pre-mapping (Quick Assessment) for the Preliminary Evaluation of Work-Related Stress

Paolo Campanini
Ergonomics of Posture and Movements
International Ergonomics School (EPM-IES)

Alberto Baratti
Territorial and hospital occupational
medicine services at ASL CN 1
Ergonomics of Posture and Movements
International Ergonomics School (EPM-IES)

CONTENTS

8.1 INTRODUCTION

The preliminary evaluation of work-related stress risk could become mandatory (almost in European Countries) because the specificity of this risk and the legislation governing it assume that the *hazard of work-related stress* is potentially present in all workplaces, regardless of the type of work or the way it is organized. Given that work-related stress is reported in all work environments, the analysis starts with the second level of pre-mapping ("Quick Assessment"): to embark on the study with excessively simple key-enters to verify the presence of this hazard is of little use.

What makes the pre-mapping work sheet for work-related stress distinctive is the outcome it generates. The various parts of the form (i.e. work content and context as risk factors reported by the homogeneous group; sentinel events associated with stress, based on information provided by the employer) not only make it possible to identify the extent of work-related stress risk and compare it with other risks but also to obtain a preliminary assessment, in compliance with some national EU regulations.

This chapter indicates how to gather the information required and fill in the work sheet and provides a few application examples.

8.2 GATHERING INFORMATION ABOUT THE HOMOGENEOUS GROUP

As for other risk factors, the information to be entered into the work sheet must be gathered by listening to the homogeneous group of workers or, if the group is too large, a few of its members in their capacity as *qualified witnesses,* i.e. workers who have a good understanding of the work and the psychosocial working environment of the homogeneous group and are able to provide a detailed description of it. A separate pre-mapping work sheet must be used for each homogeneous group of workers.

The first step is to put together a small group of workers (no more than 12). After explaining the purpose of the assessment and making it clear that its focus is on the work carried out by the homogeneous group and not their level of satisfaction with the work, the various parts of the work sheet are presented, and questions are asked to which the workers must respond by describing the daily work.

Since this is a process to collect information on the daily work performed by the homogeneous group and not a survey to gather opinions or gauge job satisfaction, the size of the group does not need to be statistically representative; it can involve only a few people who can be defined as *qualified witnesses.* Those responsible for organizing the work should oversee selecting *qualified witnesses.* The type of information that is acquired has little or no impact on workers selected as qualified witnesses.

Asking a group of qualified witnesses for information is particularly useful for obtaining a description of what really happens in the workplace, regardless of how it is formally set up. Meeting with a group of qualified witnesses should not be a cause for concern, as the information they are asked to provide is generally of an objective nature.

During the discussion the various members of the group quickly come up with a description that the majority can agree upon. Even if there are differences of opinion within the group, the exchange of ideas between the qualified witnesses will lead to a generally accepted description. The group discussion will automatically generate a single realistic description of the working conditions.

In the event of sharp disagreements, qualified witnesses must be urged to reach a single shared description; and if opinions differ widely, it will be necessary to indicate the description that represents the worst-case scenario: in this way, the rating will be more conservative, i.e. even in event of an error, the assessment will ensure the maximum protection of workers' health.

A summary of the method for reporting the information can be found in the first part of the work sheet (Figure 8.1), in addition to re-proposing the data concerning the homogeneous group acquired in the initial work sheet of the ERGOCHECK pre-mapping software.

QUICK ASSESSMENT of work-related stress

curated by Daniela Colombini, Paolo Campanini, Alberto Baratti

COMPANY NAME		Homogeneous job or group:	
Industry		Nr. of workers: Males	
		Females	

WORK SHEET 6: Quick Pre-assessment of work-related stress

INTRODUCTION The results of this pre-mapping exercise will indicate the priority and detail required to carry out a preliminary assessment of the risk of work-related stress, ALSO BASED ON THE PRIORITIES THAT EMERGED FOR ALL OTHER RISK FACTORS.
As indicated by the Framework Agreement on work-related stress of 8 October 2004 (cited in Italian Leg. Decree nr. 81/08) "stress can potentially affect any workplace and any worker, irrespective of the size of the company, field of activity, or form of employment contract or relationship". Consequently stress must be assessed in all workplaces, including small businesses.

INSTRUCTIONS FOR COMPLETING THE WORK SHEET
The form should be completed by collecting information about all or part of the homogenous group of workers and the tasks they perform. A homogenous group is defined as *"workers assigned to perform the same tasks, in the same environment (or similar), with the same working hours (or similar) and the same work organization"*.
The work sheet is broken down into SUBJECTS. For each subject there are BLOCKS of REPLIES describing scenarios that may or may not accurately depict the actual work carried out by the homogenous group.
For each SUBJECT it is necessary to provide a description that best represents the situation of the homogeneous group. For other SUBJECTS there are simple closed-ended questions.
PROVIDE ONLY ONE REPLY PER BLOCK.

FIGURE 8.1 Introduction to the work sheet relating to work-related stress.

8.3 GENERAL METHOD FOR ENTERING DATA

The pre-mapping process for assessing work-related stress risk is based on the descriptions that the homogeneous group provides on the various topics related to the type of work and working environment.

For each topic, there are blocks of answers containing different descriptors of the working environment. Based on the information reported by the homogeneous group, the answer/descriptor must be entered that best depicts the scenario presented by the group itself.

In order to more easily acquire the necessary information from the group, under the heading of each topic, there are a few examples of key questions that serve as guidelines to encourage the group to speak up on that topic. Of course, during discussions with the group, other questions can be asked, and additional details can be requested, to identify which answers/descriptors are the most appropriate, i.e. which answer/descriptor most effectively represents what is reported.

As a rule, the reference period to be analyzed is the two previous years. If the homogeneous group has been employed for less than 2 years, then the analysis should cover the period since the start of the activity.

Evaluators should always keep the reference time frame uppermost in their mind and, in case of doubt, double check with the homogeneous group; in fact, from time to time, the groups report a specific situation or event without specifying when they occurred, or refer to periods prior to the previous 2 years. If a condition or situation is reported that took place prior to the reference period, it should be disregarded.

The replies/descriptors are listed from the best to the worst situation. When selecting a reply/descriptor, all the conditions must be satisfied, otherwise the next reply/descriptor must be checked.

The evaluator's skill lies in identifying the closest reply/descriptor to the situation reported by the homogeneous group. For this, the evaluator only needs to understand the various replies and what they mean in this pre-mapping exercise. In the next section, the meaning of each reply/descriptor is provided to help the evaluator properly complete this pre-mapping section.

8.4 DESCRIPTION OF WORK CONTENT AND CONTEXT

8.4.1 WORKING ENVIRONMENT, EQUIPMENT AND TOOLS

The first subject concerns the working environment, equipment and tools (Figure 8.2). The time frame is always the previous 2 years, with some rare exceptions that are always clearly indicated. The questions do not seek to determine whether the factors considered are compliant with laws or regulations, but whether the homogeneous group considers the working environment, equipment and tools to be suitable for performing the work, effective for achieving their work objectives and not harmful to human health. The replies/descriptors refer to the following possible situations:

1. The group, or some of its members, are aware of actions to improve the physical and working environment, and equipment or tools are maintained/ renewed by the organization, so they are always in good working order. This is the ideal situation.
2. The physical working environment, equipment and tools do not cause recurring problems and the group, or some of its members, are aware of future improvements to be implemented in the short term.

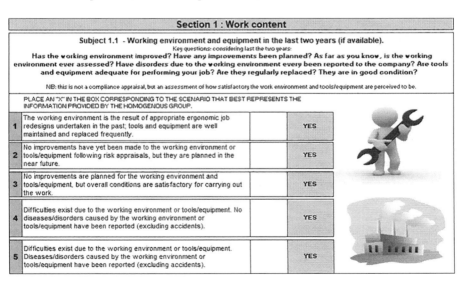

Section 1 : Work content

Subject 1.1 - Working environment and equipment in the last two years (if available).
Key questions: considering last the two years:
Has the working environment improved? Have any improvements been planned? As far as you know, is the working environment ever assessed? Have disorders due to the working environment every been reported to the company? Are tools and equipment adequate for performing your job? Are they regularly replaced? They are in good condition?

NB: this is not a compliance appraisal, but an assessment of how satisfactory the work environment and tools/equipment are perceived to be.

PLACE AN "X" IN THE BOX CORRESPONDING TO THE SCENARIO THAT BEST REPRESENTS THE INFORMATION PROVIDED BY THE HOMOGENOUS GROUP.

1	The working environment is the result of appropriate ergonomic job redesigns undertaken in the past; tools and equipment are well maintained and replaced frequently.	YES
2	No improvements have yet been made to the working environment or tools/equipment following risk appraisals, but they are planned in the near future.	YES
3	No improvements are planned for the working environment and tools/equipment, but overall conditions are satisfactory for carrying out the work.	YES
4	Difficulties exist due to the working environment or tools/equipment. No diseases/disorders caused by the working environment or tools/equipment have been reported (excluding accidents).	YES
5	Difficulties exist due to the working environment or tools/equipment. Diseases/disorders caused by the working environment or tools/equipment have been reported (excluding accidents).	YES

FIGURE 8.2 Responses/descriptors relating to the *work environment, equipment and tools.*

3. The workers are not aware of any improvements, but the working conditions, equipment or tools do not prevent them from working and achieving their work objectives.

4. There are difficulties due to the working environment, equipment or tools that prevent the workers from achieving their daily work objectives, such as: lack of adequate maintenance stopping or slowing down work and generating difficulties even for third parties (customers, patients, co-workers), use of obsolete tools or equipment that prevent prompt responses, etc.

5. In addition to what is described in point 4, workers are informed of any reports of disorders among co-workers in the last 2 years due to the work environment, equipment or tools. In this answer, it does not matter whether an actual report has been filed, but it is an indirect way of assessing whether there is a perception of a hazardous working environment, equipment or tools.

8.4.2   WORKLOAD AND WORK PACE

This topic is set out in two blocks of questions, one concerning the workload, i.e. the amount of work to be performed, and one concerning the work pace, i.e. the rate at which the work must be performed.

The first block (Figure 8.3) concerns the work pace; an assessment of work pace involves analyzing whether workers can interrupt their daily duties at their own discretion and decide when to speed up or slow down their pace. The replies/descriptors refer to the following possible situations:

1. For more than half of the working time, workers can interrupt their duties at their own discretion and decide whether to speed up their pace at given times, while still respecting the work schedule.

2. The work pace is constrained by the way the work is organized (e.g. assembly lines) or by its characteristics (e.g. customer flow and mandatory daily

Subject 1.2 - Workload and pace of work.
Key questions: for most of the shift (typically more than half of the shift)
Is the work pace pre-set (based on procedures, machinery, equipment, customer flows, deadlines)? Can the work be interrupted at the worker's discretion, for coffee or to have a break? Can the worker decide how fast to work during the shift (e.g. perform certain jobs faster or slower)?

PLACE AN "X" IN THE BOX CORRESPONDING TO THE SCENARIO THAT BEST REPRESENTS THE INFORMATION PROVIDED BY THE HOMOGENEOUS GROUP.

1 Generally speaking, workers can decide their own work pace.		YES
2 The work pace is pre-set but not rigidly (e.g. tasks on work benches and/or assembly lines with "stop and go" function; user/customer flows can be controlled; deadlines can be managed), and/or allowance is made for physiological recovery (e.g. toilet breaks, coffee) during the shift.		YES
3 The work pace is rigidly pre-set (i.e. for work on work benches and/or assembly lines, determined by user/customer flows, by pre-established response or production schedules, etc.), and/or no allowance is made for physiological recovery during the shift.		YES

FIGURE 8.3   Responses/descriptors relating to the *work pace*.

deadlines), nonetheless the set-up still allows workers to interrupt their daily duties at their own discretion and decide on the speed of execution for at least half of the working time.

3. For more than half of the working time, the work pace is constrained by the way the work is organized (e.g. assembly lines) or by requirements that prevent the workers from interrupting their activities at their own discretion for a short break because they have to be satisfied immediately, leaving no possibility to regulate the speed of execution.

The second block (Figure 8.4) concerns the workload and the question is indirect, i.e. it does not investigate the level of the workload but it is assumed that the workload increases when the hours required to cope with demand are higher than those normally agreed upon with the employer. It is important to note whether the homogeneous group includes many part-time workers, who may work "overtime" in order to take home higher wages. In this case, "overtime" should be considered as work exceeding 8 hours. The replies/descriptors refer to the following possible situations:

1. Generally speaking, the members of the homogeneous group can keep to the working hours agreed upon with the employer. They may report examples of individual workers staying on the job even after the end of their regular working hours, but most workers belonging to the homogeneous group do not. Special circumstances may also require staying on after hours, but this is an exception and is recognized as such.

2. It is almost always necessary to work one extra hour per week in order to cope with demand. This situation is widespread (i.e. involves most workers) and constant (i.e. occurs most weeks).

3. Once or twice a week (on average), the job requires putting in at least 1 hour more than the working hours agreed upon with the employer. This condition is widespread among the members of the homogeneous group and occurs almost every week.

4. More than twice a week (on average), the job requires putting in at least 1 hour more than the working hours agreed upon with the employer. This condition

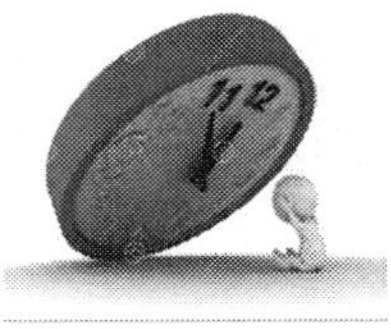

FIGURE 8.4   Responses/descriptors relating to the *work load*.

is widespread among the members of the homogeneous group and occurs almost every week. This description refers to organizations where the corporate culture deems it normal to put in extra hours or work long hours.

8.4.3 WORKING HOURS

This topic concerns the way working hours are structured (Figure 8.5). More specifically, it is interesting to know whether there is any flexibility in clocking on and off work and whether there is shift work or night shifts. These considerations also include being on call (not only as per the relevant employment contract but also unofficially, i.e. on-call via new technologies, whereby the employee feels obliged to deal with issues outside working hours). The replies/descriptors refer to the following possible situations:

1. The first condition is one of considerable flexibility in terms of clocking on and off without needing to be on-call either officially or unofficially.
2. Employees work office hours with at least some flexibility in terms of clocking on and off (at least 15 minutes' leeway), and there is no need to be on-call officially or unofficially.
3. This reply/descriptor should be checked if one of the following two situations are present: working hours are not flexible or, regardless of working hours, workers are officially on-call but can generally deal with issues remotely (on-site solutions are the exception) or, workers are unofficially on call, i.e. employees are contacted frequently (several times a week) outside working hours by phone or email and need to work at those times to deal with issues.
4. Here too only one of the following two conditions needs to be present: either there is shift work without night shifts, or employees are on-call officially or unofficially and need to be ready return to the workplace, which happens quite frequently (on average once per on-call rotation).
5. There is shift work including night shifts. No need to indicate on-call rotations.

Subject 1.3. - Working hours		
Key questions: How are working hours organized? Are there flexible working hours? Is there shift work? Are there night shifts? Are workers required to be on call?		
PLACE AN "X" IN THE BOX CORRESPONDING TO THE SCENARIO THAT BEST REPRESENTS THE INFORMATION PROVIDED BY THE HOMOGENEOUS GROUP.		
1 There are office hours or a single daily shift, but there is flexitime (workers can decide when to work).	YES	
2 There are office hours or a single daily shift with some flexibility (15-30 minutes' leeway at the beginning and end of the shift).	YES	
3 There are office hours or a single daily shift without any flexibility at the beginning or end of the shift (workers clock on and off).	YES	
4 There are several daily shifts but no night shift and/or workers are on call.	YES	
5 There are several daily shifts and also a night shift.	YES	

FIGURE 8.5 Responses/descriptors relating to the *working hours*.

8.4.4 Contact with Human Suffering

This topic should only be addressed if the work involves contact with people who are potentially in pain physically, emotionally or socially. The aim is to identify how long such contact lasts, on average, on a typical working day. The frequency scale is based on a half-day marker, i.e. whether contact lasts more or less than half a working day (Figure 8.6).

8.4.5 Contact with Users

This section is designed to assess whether difficult conditions are present due to requests received from users within or outside the organization (Figure 8.7). This does not refer to random requests from co-workers or people outside the organization that do not pertain to the job in question, but only requests from co-workers (such as human resources/staff management, technical support or front office) to solve problems.

In cases such as those mentioned above, it is necessary to assess how often the worker is required to handle requests from basic users to deal with issues that are difficult to solve. If the frequency is more than "a few times a week", i.e. practically daily, for more than half of the working hours (response 5 in the first block), the frequency with which complex or difficult requests from users are addressed must be checked, as in the examples provided for the key questions in Figure 8.7.

FIGURE 8.6 Responses/descriptors relating to *contact with suffering*.

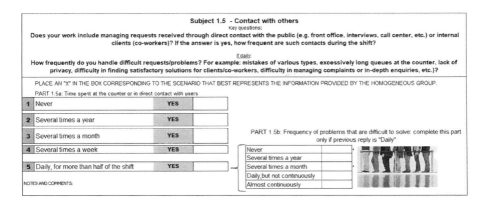

FIGURE 8.7 Responses/descriptors relating to *contact with users*.

8.4.6   RISK OF AGGRESSION

The risk of aggression must be analyzed if, over the previous 2 years, there have been cases of robbery or aggression (Figure 8.8).

The replies/descriptors refer to the following possible situations:

1. The activity does not expose workers to the risk of aggression or robbery. An example might be a back-office job without any contact with the public and no handling of money or valuables.
2. The activity might expose workers to the risk of aggression but so far nothing has ever happened.
3. As before, however, the qualified witnesses report concerns about their safety in the work place.
4. During the past 2 years at least one case of robbery or aggression was reported involving a member of the homogeneous group.
5. During the past 2 years more than one case of robbery or aggression was reported involving a member of the homogeneous group.

8.4.7   INDEPENDENT DECISION-MAKING

This section includes two blocks of questions that both refer to independent decision-making. The first block concerns the possibility of managing the workload to suit the worker's needs, and the second block concerns the possibility of using existing skills and learning new ones.

The first block (Figure 8.9) asks whether, while abiding by the organization's rules, the worker can autonomously decide on the sequence in which to perform the tasks to be carried out and how they should be performed. The replies/descriptors refer to the following possible situations:

1. Workers can decide how to perform most of their tasks, provided the rules of the organization are respected, i.e. workers can modify the way the task is performed using their own approach, strategy and method. In addition,

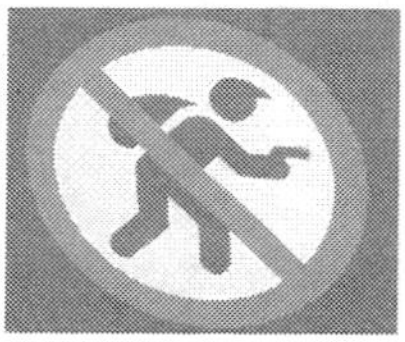

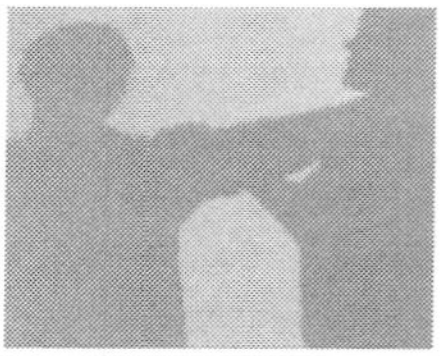

FIGURE 8.8   Responses/descriptors relating to the *risk of aggression*.

2. Work context		
Subject 2.1. - Control Key questions: Can you decide how to perform your duties, provided you abide by the rules? Are you free to decide the order in which you perform your duties?		
PLACE AN "X" IN THE BOX CORRESPONDING TO THE SCENARIO THAT BEST REPRESENTS THE INFORMATION PROVIDED BY THE HOMOGENEOUS GROUP		
1 Can you decide how to organize most of your workload, in accordance with the rules and your targets?	YES	
2 Can you decide how to organize some duties but not others, in accordance with the rules and your targets?	YES	
3 Most duties are strictly scheduled and do not allow for any personal decisions	YES	

FIGURE 8.9 Responses/descriptors relating to independent decision-making.

workers can decide the sequence in which the activities are carried out during working hours.

2. Only very few tasks can be "customized" as described above. Most activities, i.e. those taking up more than half of the working day, due to constraints such as scheduling, working methods, equipment/machinery or other reasons, cannot be personalized in terms of sequence and/or mode of execution.
3. Almost all the tasks performed during the working day are rigidly predetermined in terms of scheduling and/or working methods. Workers have little or no control over how they perform their work.

The second block of questions concerns acquiring and using work skills. The replies/descriptors refer to the following possible situations (Figure 8.10):

1. Compared to the previous 2 years, most of the group felt that they had learned new skills, and that they had improved the way they performed their tasks.
2. There have been no changes in the work over the previous 2 years, allowing workers to improve or expand their skills. The members of the group do not report any developments, nor do they report any challenges or the need to improve or expand their skills.
3. The workers in the group report a widespread need to acquire new skills or enhance existing ones, but the conditions do not allow it (e.g. lack of resources). This situation is generating several complaints and grievances about difficulties in performing the work or coping with changes.

Key questions: Does the job entail constantly learning something new, or is it always the same repetitive activity (considering the last two years)? Was useful education/training provided regarding how to cope with daily duties? Over the years have your skills and capabilities grown?		
PLACE AN "X" IN THE BOX CORRESPONDING TO THE SCENARIO THAT BEST REPRESENTS THE INFORMATION PROVIDED BY THE HOMOGENEOUS GROUP		
1 The job requires and allows for learning new skills and capabilities.	YES	
2 The job does not call for existing skills to be enhanced.	YES	
3 The job would call for continuous learning, but the conditions do not allow for new skills to be acquired or existing skills to be enhanced.	YES	

FIGURE 8.10 Responses/descriptors relating to the use of work skills.

8.4.8 Interpersonal Relations in the Workplace

This section of questions does not intend to probe the quality of interpersonal relations in the workplace, a subject that would require very different techniques for gathering information, based on an analysis of the perceptions of all the workers included in the homogeneous group. The aim is simply to verify whether there are any indicators suggesting potential interpersonal stressors within the homogeneous group. The indicators used here refer to the monitoring of relations by the organization and checking for the presence of conflicts above and beyond those regarded as "physiological" within the working population (Figure 8.11).

The replies/descriptors refer to the following possible situations:

1. The organization periodically monitors interpersonal relations through measures designed to improve them (e.g. training courses on workplace relations, conflict management, surveys and other ways of assessing the quality of relations between workers). Moreover, no interpersonal clashes have been reported in the last 2 years that have required the intervention of the organization, but minor conflicts are settled between the parties involved or with the support of their superiors.
2. There are no signs that the organization is monitoring interpersonal relations, but there have been no interpersonal conflicts in the last 2 years that have required the intervention of third parties, only the involvement of the direct superior of the clashing workers who, however, had to step in and make decisions to resolve the conflict.
3. The members of the homogeneous group report at least one case of interpersonal conflict that required the intervention of third parties in order to resolve the situation.

Subject 2.2. - Interpersonal relationships

Key questions:

Do you know if assessments are carried out that also include evaluating interpersonal relationships between co-workers and superiors? Are there any activities in place designed to improve interpersonal relationships between workers? In the last two years within your homogeneous group have there been cases of interpersonal conflicts that required the company to take action (e.g. verbal or written warnings, fines, legal action) ?

PLACE AN "X" IN THE BOX CORRESPONDING TO THE SCENARIO THAT BEST REPRESENTS THE INFORMATION PROVIDED BY THE HOMOGENEOUS GROUP.

1	•The company has put in place plans or training courses to manage workplace relationships (e.g. effective communications, teamwork, etc.) or periodically evaluates the working environment. •There have been no interpersonal conflicts that have required the company to take action.		YES
2	There have been no interpersonal conflicts requiring the company to take action (e.g. verbal or written warnings, fines, legal action) but only the intervention of a superior (e.g. area manager, department head, shift manager, office manager, etc.).		YES
3	There has been at least one case of interpersonal conflict (in the last two years) that has called for the company to take action (e.g. verbal or written warnings, fines, legal action) or a case of mobbing.		YES

Key questions:

Are there any activities that entail working in isolation (such as to cause distress)? If so, does this last for more than half of the shift?

1	The job calls for physical isolation (such as to cause distress) for over half of the shift		YES		NO

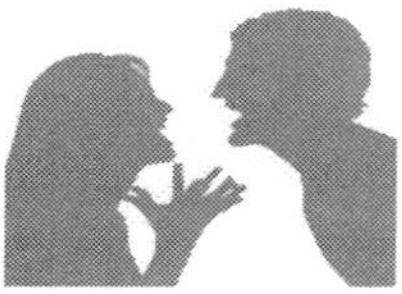

FIGURE 8.11 Responses/descriptors relating to interpersonal relations.

Lastly, there is a single section for reporting the presence of workplace isolation, i.e. when there are no face-to-face communications with co-workers for more than half of the daily working hours. This condition must occur almost daily and must be described by the group as a critical condition.

8.4.9 Work–Life Balance

Although this section refers to aspects that do not pertain exclusively to the workplace, and by definition, include situations falling outside the working environment, it is nevertheless interesting to assess this specific risk, as it has a recognized impact on work-related stress.

The main points considered concern the general willingness of the homogeneous group's superiors/supervisors to manage the work–life balance of their subordinates, and the possible presence of widespread complaints within the homogeneous group regarding their work–life balance (Figure 8.12)

The replies/descriptors refer to the following possible situations:

1. The first reply/descriptor defines working conditions in which both elements are present: on the one hand, the commitment of superiors/supervisors to manage the work–life balance of their subordinates is recognized; and on the other hand, the organization has put in place activities or services that seek to improve the work–life balance of its workers.
2. The second reply/descriptor only considers whether superiors/supervisors are prepared to manage the work–life balance of their subordinates.
3. The third reply/descriptor indicates conditions in which there are no specific widespread problems in reconciling work and life, but no attention is paid to the issue. Benefits are those provided for by law and granted at the request of the individual worker experiencing difficulties.
4. The fourth option indicates that there are no widespread problems and that the organization and superiors/supervisors do not pay attention to the work–life balance.

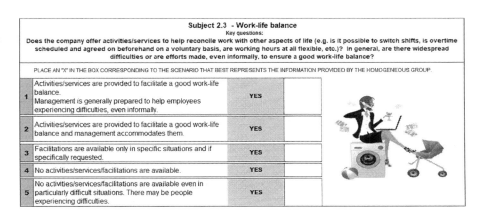

FIGURE 8.12 Responses/descriptors relating to the possibility of reconciling work and life.

5. The last reply/descriptor specifically refers to widespread difficulties in finding a suitable work–life balance, i.e. workers report more than one instance when it has been difficult to reconcile personal or family commitments with work demands.

8.4.10 Possibility to Report Harassment and/or Abuse in the Workplace

This section is designed to assess whether some or all the workers belonging to the homogeneous group are aware of the possibility to report abuse or harassment at work (Figure 8.13). Finding out whether they know how to report such situations is less important than discovering if they are familiar with company systems or procedures and know who to turn to in the company in the event of distress due to abuse or harassment. If any of these conditions are present, then it is necessary to indicate "Yes". It is not possible to indicate 'Yes' if the workers indicate that the only solution is to take their complaints outside the organization, such as to a trade union or other external organization.

8.5 COMPLETING THE SECTION ON SENTINEL EVENTS

Figure 8.14 shows the final table to be completed in order to define so-called "sentinel events". The information must be obtained from the employer and refers to the homogeneous group in question, regarding the last 3 years.

The blank spaces in the table should be checked (with an "X") if the situation described in the first line of the table is present. To complete this part on sentinel events, it is preferable to base the responses on numerical indexes calculated on real data: if precise data is unavailable, at least the "perception of the event" provided by the homogeneous group can be reported.

8.5.1 Potentially Stress-Related Occupational Disorders/Diseases

The first question concerns the presence (over the last 3 years) of occupational disorders/diseases related to work-related stress, as reported and notified to the company and recognized by the national INAIL – the Italian Institute for Insurance against Accidents at Work).

Subject 2.4 - Possibility to report harassment and abuse
Key questions:
Are procedures/guidelines in place for reporting abuse or harassment by superiors or co-workers?

NB: please reply to each separate question in this block

if you are aware of these circumstances please reply, otherwise leave blank:

1	There are procedures/guidelines in place for reporting abuse or harassment and employees are informed of them.	YES	
		NO	

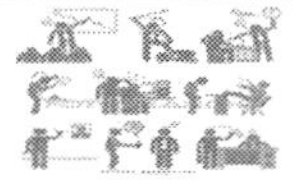

FIGURE 8.13 Responses/descriptors relating to the possibility of reporting harassment or abuse in the workplace.

3. Hazard (signs that may indicate a problem of work related stress)				
Subject 3.1 Data available from the company on safety, sickness and disciplinary action, as effects of work-related stress (This data must be requested from the company) *Fill in with company data: requested data and trends calculated over the last 3 years: if non available, leave the box blank.*				
	PRESENCE OF THE EVENT LEAVE BLANK IF NONE, MARK WITH AN "X" IF PRESENT	INCREASE IN THE EVENT reported over the last 3 years LEAVE BLANK IF NONE,	EVENT HIGHER THAN THE COMPANY AVERAGE more frequent than the company average	DESCRIPTIVE NUMERICAL DATA Enter any specific quantitative/numerical data that may be available (e.g. number of events, frequency, etc.) and the relevant year.
1 Work-related diseases/disorders caused by occupational stress certified by a physician (LEAVE THE BOX BLANK IF NONE)				
1 Turnover (resignations)				
1 Disciplinary actions				
1 Medical examination requested by the worker				
1 Sick leave				
1 Occupational injuries (not on-going)				

FIGURE 8.14 Table for defining sentinel events or company data.

The box should only be checked if, in the previous 3 years, there were any reports of occupational disorders/diseases caused by or related to occupational stress. This information is easily available from the employer. If there are no reports of occupational disorders/diseases due to a stressful working environment, the box remains blank.

8.5.2 Voluntary Resignations

The second line requires the evaluator to calculate the number of voluntary resignations during the last 3 years in the homogeneous group, and to observe trends. The best way to evaluate voluntary resignations is to calculate an index for the ratio of resignations to the number of members of the homogeneous group, i.e. the number of resignations is taken as the numerator and the number of people in the homogeneous group as the denominator. The index of voluntary resignations is obtained by multiplying the result by 100.

It is possible to calculate trends for this data over the 3-year period, as well as for the following data, by comparing the figure for the previous year with the average for the 3 years taken into consideration. If the figure for the previous year is higher than the average, then it will be necessary to check the "increase of the event" box; if it is equal or less, then the box will remain blank.

The "event above the company average" box should be checked only if the figure for the previous year is higher than the same figure considering the entire employee population (which also includes the homogeneous group) and not the homogeneous group on its own.

All these important figures can be saved in the last column on the right (DESCRIPTIVE NUMERICAL DATA) of the table in Figure 8.14.

8.5.3 DISCIPLINARY EVENTS

This box should only be checked if any formal disciplinary measures have been taken (complaints, written or verbal warnings, etc.) against any member of the homogeneous group in the last 3 years.

8.5.4 MEDICAL EXAMINATION REQUESTED BY THE WORKER

Workers may request a medical examination with the designated physician to verify if the job is compatible with their health. This section reports on such requests. As with voluntary resignations, it is advisable to create an index that considers the number of requests for medical examinations in relation to the number of members of the homogeneous group and multiply the result by 100.

The "increase in the event" box must be checked if the figure for the previous year is higher than the average for the 3-year period under consideration. Conversely, the "event above the company average" box should be checked only if the figure for the previous year is higher than the same figure for the entire employee population (also including the homogeneous group) and not the homogeneous group on its own.

8.5.5 SICK LEAVE

Here too, the creation of an index would be the ideal way to calculate the trend for the 3-year period and compare the previous year with the overall average for the working population in the company.

Calculating the days (or hours) of sick leave means not considering any absences other than the worker's illness, such as maternity leave, sick children, etc.

The index to be worked out may relate to sick leave in relation to the number of days (or hours) that the worker can perform or with respect to the number of workers in the homogeneous group.

As in the case of the other indicators, evaluators will check the boxes for absences due to illness only if the absences of the previous year are higher than the average of the 3 years in question and higher than the average for the whole working population.

8.5.6 ACCIDENTS

Workplace accidents have generally already been calculated and the indexes referring to them are usually available. In this case, it would be ideal to consider only accidents that occurred in the workplace. As for the other indexes, the evaluator should evaluate the trend over the 3-year period, i.e. whether the figure for the previous year is higher than the 3-year average, and whether the figure for the homogeneous group for the previous year is higher than the average for the entire working population.

8.6 CRITERIA FOR CALCULATING SCORES AND CALCULATION METHOD

8.6.1 CALCULATION OF *EXPOSURE LEVEL* USING DATA FROM THE HOMOGENEOUS GROUP

This section of the ERGOCHECK program involves asking the homogeneous group of workers (or the group of qualified witnesses) to describe their tasks in relation to a series of specific psychosocial factors. For each of these factors, the description that most closely follows that reported by the group involved and indicated in the checklist is identified.

Once the checklist is completed, a calculation algorithm based on the "Job Demands Resources" model (Bakker and Demerouti, 2007; 2017), described in Chapter 2.3, produces a numerical result that identifies the exposure level as "optimal", "acceptable", "medium", "high" or "critical". The exposure level is calculated based on the score for each description of each checklist item. The Job Demands Resources model identifies not only the job demands but also any resources that may favorably affect the relationship between job demands and the condition ("strain") associated with them. The score assigned to the selected descriptions is used to determine both the risk exposure level, by identifying potentially high work-related stress (increasing the final score), and the efforts to reduce risk exposure, in cases where the checked description includes a "condition" supporting the work (linked to values that reduce the score).

Lastly, each psychosocial factor detected through the descriptions is differently weighted (*Multiplier*) (Figure 8.15) in the calculation of the final score. The value of the multiplier is determined based on the strength of the relationship between the psychosocial factor that determines potential work-related stress and the health outcomes.

By applying the different *Multipliers* to the individual *factor scores*, the *exposure score for the individual factor* can be calculated: adding all the scores thus obtained for each individual factor produces the final score.

The lowest values indicate optimal general working conditions or job demands that are satisfactorily offset by the number of employees present (i.e. workplace well-being). The highest scores on the rating scale indicate a more challenging work environment. In practice, as the score increases, so does the potential for exposure to work-related stress.

The results do not show the final score but rather, following a breakdown of the range of possible scores (from 0 to 40), the category in which the score falls. The classification of the results into categories is based on an empirical observation of working conditions in relation to the results obtained:

- Scores from 0 to 9.2 (23% of the scale) indicate that work-related stress exposure is "optimal", and indicative of well-being in the work place.
- Scores from 9.2 to 19 indicate that workers are exposed to "acceptable" conditions, i.e. conditions that require a limited amount of effort to be sustained (24%–47%).

No.questions	Scores	Multipliers	No.questions	Scores	Multipliers
Subject 1.1 Working environment, equipment			Subject 1.6 Risk of violence or aggression		
1	0	1	1	0	1
2	1	1	2	1	1
3	1	1	3	2	1
4	2	1	4	2	1
5	3	1	5	2	1
Subject 1.2 Workload			Subject 2.1. - Control		
1	0	3	1	0	2
2	1	3	2	1	2
3	2	3	3	2	2
Subject 1.2 Pace of work.			Subject 2.1 Training		
1	0	3	1	0	1
2	1	3	2	1	1
3	2	3	3	2	1
4	2	3			
Subject 1.3 Working hours			Subject 2.2 Interpersonal relationships		
1	0	2	1	0	2
2	1	2	2	1	2
3	1	2	3	2	2
4	2	2	Subject 2.2 Working in isolation		
5	2	2	1	1	1
Subject 1.4 Contact with suffering			Subject 2.3 Work-life balance		
1	0	2	1	0	2
2	1	2	2	1	2
3	1	2	3	1	2
4	2	2	4	1	2
5	2	2	5	2	2
Subject 1.5 Contact with others			Subject 2.4 Report harassment and abuse		
5.1	0	2	1	1	1
5.2	1	2			
5.3	1	2			
5.4	2	2			
5.5	2	2			

FIGURE 8.15 Intrinsic scores and multipliers for each psychosocial factor in order to calculate exposure levels.

- Scores from 19 to 29.5 fall within the "average" exposure range; i.e. conditions that require putting constant effort into the work in order to manage it adequately (48%–73%).
- Scores from 29.5 to 38 indicate a "high" level of exposure (74%–95%).
- Scores above 38 (above 95% of the score scale) indicate "critical" exposure.

These last two conditions indicate working conditions that require continuous high psychophysical effort to manage the work.

Exposure levels can be classified into categories not only using the final scores but also specific responses that directly identify "critical" exposure levels, regardless of the quantitative result obtained. The most authoritative scientific models for occupational stress have already identified conditions that may present a risk to worker health.

Accordingly, in line with the Job Demand Control model (Karasek and Theorell, 1990), "critical" exposure will be attributed to responses that indicate:

- High workload;
- Low job control;
- Low "social support".

Other potential causes of Burnout (Maslach et al., 2001), directly defining "critical" exposure, are:

- High workload;
- Contact with troubled or suffering users.

8.6.2 CALCULATING THE *SEVERITY INDEX* THROUGH "SENTINEL EVENTS"

The "sentinel events" data also produce an index; in this case, it is a severity index. The calculation of the index considers the relationship of the data with a potentially high work-related stress situation, thus attributing a different weight (Multiplier) to the data in terms of both Scores and Multipliers (Figure 8.16). In accordance with the regulatory requirements for defining the risk of work-related stress, the data taken into consideration was selected based on its connection to work-related stress (Campanini, 2014).

The calculation of the severity index considers the sentinel events of the previous 3 years. As indicated in Section 8.5, it is advisable to create indexes for evaluating the data.

The severity index has been calculated considering three dimensions:

a. Comparative score: The score indicated in the previous figure is attributed to the sentinel event only if the previous year's score for the homogeneous group is higher than the company average for the same year. For this score, the data relating to voluntary resignations, unscheduled medical examinations, sick leave, and accidents are taken into consideration.
b. Trend score: For each sentinel event, the average for the 3-year period of the homogeneous group is compared with the score for the previous year; if the score for the last year is higher than the average of the 3-year period, a score double that of the sentinel event indicated in the previous figure is attributed. For this score, the data relating to voluntary resignations, unscheduled medical examinations, sick leave and accidents are taken into consideration.

	Scores		
	INCREASE IN THE EVENT	EVENT HIGHER THAN THE COMPANY AVERAGE	Multiplier
Work-related diseases/disorders caused by occupational stress certified by a physician (LEAVE THE BOX BLANK IF NONE)	2	1	2
Turnover (resignations)	2	1	1,5
Disciplinary actions	2	1	0,5
Medical examination requested by the worker	2	1	0,5
Sick leave	2	1	1,5
Occupational injuries (not on-going)	2	1	0,5

FIGURE 8.16 Scores and multipliers for "sentinel events" in order to calculate the severity index.

c. Presence score: For sentinel events due to reported occupational diseases related to work-related stress and disciplinary events, the score indicated in the previous figure is given only if there has been at least one event in the last 3 years.

The final score of the severity index is the sum of all the scores calculated as indicated above. A scale is thus defined that goes from 0 to 14.5 points which, through empirical evaluations, has been broken down into four levels of severity: "absent", "low", "medium" and "high":

- "absent" corresponds to 5% of the scale (lowest scores) and indicates no potential consequences deriving from work-related stress.
- "low" includes scores from 5% to 45% of the scale and indicates potential consequences deriving from work-related stress.
- Scores from 45% to 95% of the scale indicate likely consequences deriving from work-related stress risk and are classified as "medium".
- Scores that include the upper 5% of the scale are classified as "high" and indicate the presence of consequences due to the potential risk of work-related stress.

8.7   FINAL OVERALL RESULTS

Once completed, the work sheet produces three separate results:

- The first result relates directly to the content and context part of the analysis but does not consider the company data (sentinel events). The result obtained with the information provided directly by the workers belonging to the homogeneous group flows into the summary section, defining the level of priority of work-related stress risk compared to other risks (Chapter 9). If a summary is all that is required, all that needs to be filled in are the sections on job content and context without checking the sentinel events.
- The second result is the visual depiction of the most critical factors via the radar graph (Figure 8.17). As before, to obtain this result all that is needed is to fill in the content and context part of the analysis. The graph shows which of the factor has the greatest influence on exposure to work-related stress. The factors with the highest percentages therefore represent the largest area of the graph that are the top-priority factors to be addressed in order to put in place corrective or compensatory measures in relation to work-related stress.
- Lastly, if the entire work sheet is completed, i.e. job content, context and sentinel events, it is possible to generate a preliminary assessment of the risk of work-related stress. The outcome produced by completing the whole work sheet consists in a risk matrix (Figure 8.18) that on the horizontal axis indicates the level of exposure to stressful factors on the basis of work context and content (classified into five levels: "optimal", "acceptable",

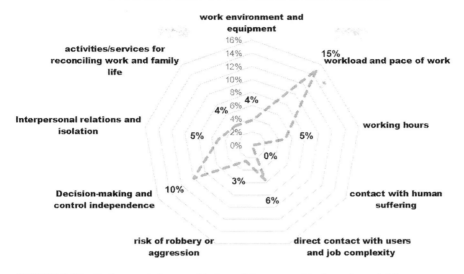

FIGURE 8.17   Radar graph for a rapid view of the most critical psychosocial factors.

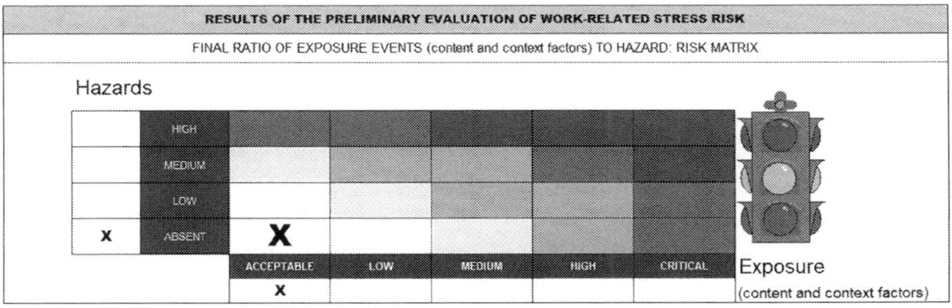

FIGURE 8.18   Risk matrix for defining work-related stress levels.

"medium", "high" and "critical") and, on the vertical axis, the severity index based on company data or the analysis of sentinel events (classified into four levels: "negligible", "low", "medium" and "high").

Figure 8.18 shows that by crossing exposure levels with severity levels, different overall risk levels are obtained, i.e. from risk "absent" changing to "critical" risk, and with "traffic light" colors providing an instant indication of the risk level:

- Risk "absent" (green) indicates optimal working condition with respect to the risk of work-related stress and may be associated with well-being in the workplace.

- "Acceptable" risk (yellow) indicates working conditions where there are elements of work-related stress that can be managed but must be monitored. This level of risk refers to a working condition that does not require the mandatory adoption of corrective or compensatory measures, although it would be advisable to put in place actions to support the welfare of workers in order to avoid potentially higher exposure going forward.
- "Medium" risk (orange) indicates working conditions that in general is associated with the risk of work-related stress, where the work demands are not adequately balanced by the workers and the working conditions include a considerable amount of activities that cannot be sustained without psychophysical effort. In this case, corrective and compensatory measures are necessary and mandatory.
- "High" risk (red) indicates working conditions featuring high stress levels, for which it is necessary and mandatory to put in place corrective and compensatory measures as a matter of urgency, in order to rapidly restore better working conditions.
- "Critical" risk indicates working conditions situated in the fifth highest percentile of the evaluation scales of the two indexes considered, i.e. extreme conditions. Only the combination of either a "high" severity index and "medium", "high" or "critical" exposure level or a "medium" or "high" severity index with a "critical" exposure level can produce "critical" risk. This level of risk indicates conditions that test the psychophysical endurance of workers and requires mandatory and urgent action to change the way the work is performed and rapidly make it ergonomically acceptable.

Figure 8.19 summarizes the meanings of the different risk levels and consequent actions.

Figure 8.20 indicates whether any of the conditions detected are critical, i.e. responses resulting in a "critical" level of exposure, as described in Section 8.6. If working conditions are critical, the boxes in this table will be colored to indicate the combination to which the critical conditions correspond to.

WORKING CONDITIONS	RESULTING ACTIONS	RISK LEVEL
OPTIMAL:	MAINTAIN current working conditions	ACCEPTABLE
BORDERLINE: manageable stressors present	SUSTAIN the situation and monitor criticalities	LOW
GENERAL WORKING CONDITIONS INVOLVE WORK-RELATED STRESS RISK	IMPROVE with corrective or compensatory measures	MEDIUM
GENERAL WORKING CONDITIONS INVOLVE HIGH WORK-RELATED STRESS RISK	RECOVER with corrective or compensatory measures, to be introduced as quickly as possible	HIGH
GENERAL WORKING CONDITIONS INVOLVE VERY HIGH WORK-RELATED STRESS RISK	ADJUST, corrective or compensatory measures are urgently required	CRITICAL

FIGURE 8.19   Summary of the meanings of the different risk levels and consequent actions.

CRITICAL SITUATIONS determined by pre-established combinations of exposure factors	CRITICAL1 (Burn-out from contact with suffering)	CRITICAL 2 (Burn-out from contact with others)	CRITICAL 3 (job-demand control, Karasek)
work environment and equipment			
workload and pace of work			
working hours			
contact with human suffering			
direct contact with others and job complexity			
risk of robbery or aggression			
independent decision-making and control			
interpersonal relationships and isolation			
activities/services for reconciling work and family life			
CRITICAL SITUATION PRESENT			

FIGURE 8.20   Summary of the presence of critical situations.

8.8   A PRACTICAL EXAMPLE OF HOW TO COMPLETE THE WORK SHEET

As described in the general introductory section of this chapter, the work sheet has been used in different work settings and in different sectors, in small and large companies, among homogeneous groups of workers identified in accordance with the relevant legislation and fully adopted in the procedures proposed herein.

More specifically, the work sheet has been tested in the health sector, both among healthcare professionals and administrative support staff, as well as in banking, foodservice, information technology and education.

The authors decided to provide a detailed example of the utilization of the pre-mapping work sheet and preliminary analysis of work-related stress via an evaluation performed in the kitchens of a large hospital.

At the time of the analysis, the company that provided this service employed about 1,200 workers in food service, storage and logistics, information technology, administration and health care at major hospitals throughout Italy's Piedmont region.

The homogeneous group, which is the subject of the evaluation presented here, is comprised of 4 men and 7 women, totaling 11 employees: their work consists in the assembly line preparation of lunch and dinner trays to be delivered to patients in the hospital wards. For lunch, an average of 690 trays are prepared in about 90 minutes (minimum 75 minutes), while for dinner, 600 trays are prepared (the number is lower than for lunch, as the Day Hospital wards are closed). The group spends the remaining working time preparing the premises and equipment, receiving supplies and, at the end of the day, cleaning the premises and equipment.

The work is performed 24/7, with shifts and breaks in accordance with employment contracts.

The organization of the work of preparing trays on an assembly line is very strict and hierarchical: nine different activities were identified, involving the use of fixed workstations, which could not be modified at the time of the assessment:

- At the first station, the operator starts and stops the assembly line at the touch of a button, and positions the empty tray with the disposable cutlery.
- Along the line, seven operators place dishes and containers with different first courses, second courses, bread, seasonings, vegetables and fruit.
- Two operators at the end of the line check that the trays are prepared properly and completely, according to the requests of the patient or dietitian; they add a water bottle and load the tray onto a meals trolley, which is closed and positioned for transportation to the various floors by the eleventh operator.

While workplace assessments were in progress utilizing the pre-mapping work sheet, due to emerging problems and organizational criticalities, the evaluation was also completed by filling in the work sheet regarding the organization of the work and work-related stress. Figure 8.21 summarizes the results of the assessment generated by pre-mapping all the work place risk factors present; the organizational and work-related stress data remain to be completed.

Below is a description of the critical issues arising from time to time in the various sections of the work sheet specifically devoted to the work organization and work-related stress, so as to complete the entire ERGOCHECK process (Figure 8.22).

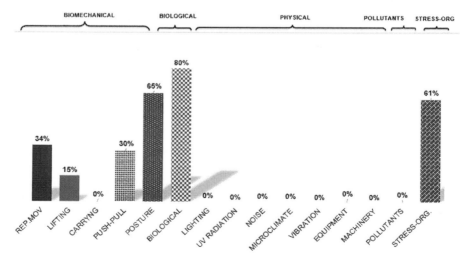

FIGURE 8.21 Preparation of meal trays on conveyor belt: results of pre-mapping for all work environment factors and for the risk of biomechanical overload.

Subject 1.1 Working environment and equipment in the last two years (if available).	

Difficulties exist due to the working environment or tools/equipment. Diseases/disorders caused by the working environment or tools/equipment have been reported (excluding accidents).

Subject 1.2 Workload and pace of work.

-The work pace is rigidly pre-set (i.e. for work on work benches and/or assembly lines, determined by user/customer flows, by pre-established response or production schedules, etc.), and/or no allowance is made for physiological recovery during the shift.
-The workload requires prolonging working hours or working overtime by up to an hour, at least once a week.

Subject 1.3 Working hours

There are several daily shifts but no night shift and/or workers are on call.

Subject 1.4 Contact with suffering

Subject 1.5 Contact with others

Daily, for more than half of the shift: Daily,but not continuously

Subject 1.6 Risk of violence or aggression

Never, since there is nothing to rob and/or no reason for an aggression.

Subject 2.1. - Control

-Most duties are strictly scheduled and do not allow for any personal decisions
-The job does not call for existing skills to be enhanced.

Subject 2.2 Interpersonal relationships

There has been at least one case of interpersonal conflict (in the last two years) that has called for the company to take action (e.g. verbal or written warnings, fines, legal action) or a case of mobbing.

Subject 2.3 Work-life balance

No activities/services/facilitations are available even in particularly difficult situations. There may be people experiencing difficulties.

Subject 2.4 Possibility to report harassment and abuse

There are procedures/guidelines in place for reporting abuse or harassment and employees are informed of them.

FIGURE 8.22 Responses given by the homogeneous group tasked with preparing trays to the questions asked in the specific work sheet with regard to work "content" and "context".

8.8.1 PART 1: WORK CONTENT

8.8.1.1 Section 1.1: Working environment, equipment and tools

As stated, this section does not intend to assess whether the physical working conditions are in accordance with rules and regulations, but more simply to determine if the homogeneous group considers the environment, equipment and tools to be suitable for the work to be performed and not harmful to their health.

In this case, most of the operators, except those at the start and end of the line, complained about being unable to rotate among the various stations, the poor organization of both the work spaces and the arrangement of the objects to be picked up and placed on the trays, which then go to the assembly line. The noisy working environment, due to the proximity of other activities, and the placement of the equipment often hinders communications between operators, with frequent misunderstandings and mistakes, causing tensions and continuous arguments between operators and anxiety in some, especially short-term or casual workers, for fear of making mistakes and being continuously reprimanded.

Reply number 5 was therefore entered.

8.8.1.2   Section 1.2: Workload and work pace

The work pace is determined by production schedules, which are very strict and unchangeable.

Workers must wait for the food to be prepared in the kitchen, then transport it on the same conveyor belt, and very quickly fill the trays and send the trolleys to all the wards and the emergency room. The assembly line rarely stops and only in the event of mistakes. During preparation (and therefore for about 75–90 minutes), it is not possible to move away from the line or be replaced.

Workers are not infrequently asked to work extra hours.

The most appropriate response is therefore no. 3 in the first box: "pace", and no. 3 in the second box: "workload".

8.8.1.3   Section 1.3: Working hours

The working hours are rigid, no flexibility is guaranteed, neither on the morning shift nor the afternoon shift.

There are no night shifts or on-call rotations.

The most appropriate response is thus no. 4.

8.8.1.4   Section 1.4: Contact with human suffering

The homogeneous group never comes into direct contact with patients or users outside the hospital.

The most appropriate response is therefore no. 1.

8.8.1.5   Section 1.5: Contact with users/patients

This section determines whether there are difficulties due to demands received from patients or users even within the same organization. Demands routinely received from co-workers, regardless of their nature, are not taken into consideration, but only those activities that expressly require the employee to take on board demands/problems from co-workers and find a solution.

The homogeneous group complained about receiving last-minute demands from the department's health care or dietitians every day, sometimes several times per shift, to prepare and deliver special meals for patients, forcing the group to contact the kitchen and discuss the preparation and wait for the food to arrive, delaying the work flow and also prolonging the working hours. Meanwhile, the ward complained about delays or mistakes.

According to the group such situations were due to the poor organization of the work and the absence of official procedures, leading to continuous arguments within the group and with co-workers in the kitchen or wards, almost always forcing them to seek last-minute solutions to address specific issues for specific patients or wards.

The most appropriate response is the combination of no. 5 and "daily but not constantly".

8.8.1.6   Section 1.6: Risk of violence/aggression

This risk was not present in the work environment examined here.

The reply is therefore no. 1.

8.8.2 PART 2: WORK CONTEXT

8.8.2.1 Section 2.1: Independent decision-making in the workplace

As mentioned, this section includes two blocks of questions that both address the presence or absence of decision-making power.

The first block determines whether the worker can tailor the work to their own needs and asks if it is possible to independently decide the sequence of the tasks to be carried out and how they are performed.

As previously stated, the group is not able to make any decisions independently or tailor the work to their needs.

The job is quite monotonous and repetitive, and in fact does not require any training, except for what is provided for by the relevant legislation with respect to exposure to ergonomic risks.

The most appropriate responses to question no. 3 are: "decision-making power", for the first box and 2: "improving skills", for the second.

8.8.2.2 Section 2.2: Interpersonal relations and workplace isolation

Interpersonal relations are extremely conflictual, and on several occasions the intervention, sometimes formal, of superiors and the company was required to deal with serious interpersonal conflicts between members of the group, or between certain members and their direct superiors, or with co-workers in the kitchen or wards, or with dietitians.

The correct response was no. 3.

No members of the group worked alone; therefore, the response to that specific question is: No.

8.8.2.3 Section 2.3: Work–life balance

Relations with employees are rigid and pre-determined; no efforts are made to facilitate a good work–life balance; therefore, the correct response is no. 4.

8.8.2.4 Section 2.4: Possibility to report harassment and abuse

In the period prior to the analysis, management had explained how to report abuse or harassment in the workplace to the person in charge and to the supervisor, so the correct answer is: YES.

8.8.3 SECTION 3: SENTINEL EVENTS

The determination of the final figure (Figure 8.24) was made possible thanks to the data provided by the company management and referred to the homogeneous group in question.

This additional objective information made it possible to complete the preliminary assessment of work-related stress for this group of workers.

No occupational diseases or disorders were reported due to work-related stress, but in recent years, there was a gradual increase in resignations, requests for medical examinations (also due to work-related distress and not only to report musculoskeletal disorders), sick leave due to sickness and accidents, at a consistently higher rate than the company average (Figure 8.23).

Subject 3.1 Data available from the company on safety, sickness and disciplinary action, as effects of work-related stress (This data must be requested from the company)

Fill in with company data: requested data and trends calculated over the last 3 years: if non available, leave the box blank.

		PRESENCE OF THE EVENT LEAVE BLANK IF NONE. MARK WITH AN "X" IF PRESENT		INCREASE IN THE EVENT reported over the last 3 years LEAVE BLANK IF NONE, MARK WITH AN "X" IF	EVENT HIGHER THAN THE COMPANY AVERAGE more frequent than the company average LEAVE BLANK IF	DESCRIPTIVE NUMERICAL DATA Enter any specific quantitative/numerical data that may be available (e.g. number of events, frequency, etc.) and the relevant year.
1	Work-related diseases/disorders caused by occupational stress certified by a physician (LEAVE THE BOX BLANK IF NONE)					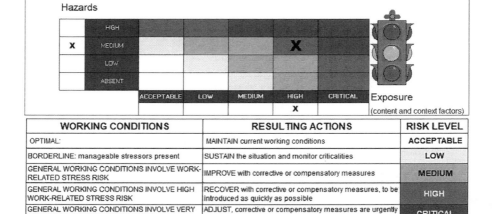
1	Turnover (resignations)			x	x	
1	Disciplinary actions					
1	Medical examination requested by the worker				x	
1	Sick leave			x	x	
1	Occupational injuries (not on-going)				x	

FIGURE 8.23 The study of sentinel events.

8.8.4 FINAL RESULTS FOR THE HOMOGENEOUS GROUP OF WORKERS TASKED WITH PREPARING TRAYS ON AN ASSEMBLY LINE

The information collected from workers with regard to the work content and context, and from the company with regard to sentinel events, has made it possible to complete the work sheet and finalize the preliminary assessment of the risk of work-related stress in this homogeneous group of workers, in accordance with Italian and European regulations.

The situation was found to be HIGH risk, calling for urgent corrective and compensatory measures in order to rapidly improve working conditions (Figure 8.24).

WORKING CONDITIONS	RESULTING ACTIONS	RISK LEVEL
OPTIMAL:	MAINTAIN current working conditions	ACCEPTABLE
BORDERLINE: manageable stressors present	SUSTAIN the situation and monitor criticalities	LOW
GENERAL WORKING CONDITIONS INVOLVE WORK-RELATED STRESS RISK	IMPROVE with corrective or compensatory measures	MEDIUM
GENERAL WORKING CONDITIONS INVOLVE HIGH WORK-RELATED STRESS RISK	RECOVER with corrective or compensatory measures, to be introduced as quickly as possible	HIGH
GENERAL WORKING CONDITIONS INVOLVE VERY HIGH WORK-RELATED STRESS RISK	ADJUST, corrective or compensatory measures are urgently required	CRITICAL

FIGURE 8.24 Result of the preliminary evaluation of work-related stress.

**DESCRIPTIVE AREAS RELATING TO PRIORITIES BASED ON REPLIES :
PERCENTAGES OF INDIVIDUAL RISK FACTORS**

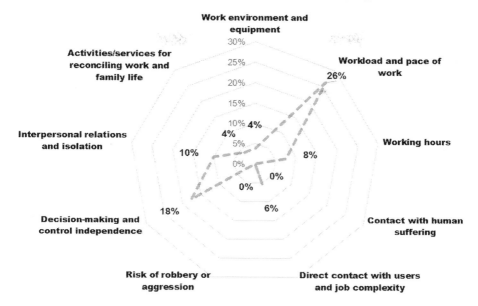

FIGURE 8.25 Result of the evaluation of the content and context sections of the analysis using radar graphs depicting the various factors examined.

Thanks to the indications generated through the work sheet, the figures depicting the results of the analysis, and the radar graph that provided a rapid view of the most critical factors (Figure 8.25), the management of the company has decided to conduct an in-depth investigation and to adopt corrective measures subject to ongoing assessments, also in light of the ergonomics-driven reorganization of the work implemented after the intervention.

8.9 EXAMPLES OF APPLICATIONS

The ERGOCHECK program for the preliminary evaluation of work-related stress has also been applied to other homogeneous groups in a variety of different jobs, work settings and markets, in order to verify its effectiveness.

The results are summarized in Table 8.1, which shows the sector in which the homogeneous group works, the name of the homogeneous group corresponding to the activity carried out by the workers, the level of exposure to work-related stress and, in the last column under the heading "Notes", a summary of the working conditions that determined the level of exposure.

Exposure levels for this specific risk may vary regardless of the task and sector involved. Although referring to similar tasks in the same sector, the application of the assessment to "food service workers" in the healthcare sector led to different levels of exposure to work-related stress ranging from "optimal" to critical linked according to the Job Demands Control stress model.

TABLE 8.1

Work Sectors and Results for Homogeneous Groups Submitted to Work Sheet Analysis

Sector	Homogeneous Group	Exposure Level	Remarks
Education	Primary school teachers	Optimal – code green	Good working conditions with well-balanced resources
Education	Cookery school teachers	Optimal – code green	Good working conditions with well-balanced resources
Care work	Educators	Acceptable – code yellow	Working conditions with satisfactory resources, but with shift work, contact with problematic users and contact with suffering
Food service	School canteen workers	Optimal – code green	Good working conditions with well-balanced resources
Health care	911 triage nurses	Critical – code purple	Critical risk of burnout. Shift work, contact with problematic users and contact with suffering
Health care	Administrative staff	Optimal – code green	Good working conditions with well-balanced resources
Chemicals	Industrial laboratory technician	Optimal – code green	Good working conditions with well-balanced resources
Health care	Administrative staff	Optimal – code green	Good working conditions with well-balanced resources
IT	IT support	Optimal – code green	Good working conditions with well-balanced resources
Health care	Food service workers	High – code red	Low decision-making power, extremely challenging work environment
Health care	Food service workers	Optimal – code green	Good working conditions with well-balanced resources
Health care	Food service workers	Optimal – code green	Good working conditions with well-balanced resources
Health care	Food service workers	Optimal – code green	Good working conditions with well-balanced resources
Health care	Food service workers	Critical – code purple	Critical working conditions (Job Demand Control model)
Health care	Specialist in forensic medicine	High – code red	High work load and difficult personal relations
Health care	Nurses – forensic medicine	Medium – code orange	Contact with users presenting complex issues
Health care	Outpatient clinic nurses	Critical – code purple	Critical risk of burnout: high work load, contact with problematic users and difficult interpersonal relations
Health care	Radiologist	Critical – code purple	Critical working conditions (Job Demand Control model)
Food service	Workers in highway diners	Optimal – code green	Good working conditions with well-balanced resources
Banking services	Bank staff, financial services	Critical – code purple	High work load, shift work, contact with problematic users, increased sick leave

This is understandable since the work sheet assesses, as objectively as possible, the psychosocial working conditions that, regardless of the sector or the specific task, can vary significantly. Thus, while in some situations there are optimal working conditions, i.e. acceptable workloads and satisfactory work resources, in others the workloads are extremely high and there are no specific resources, and elsewhere workers have little decision-making power and there are interpersonal conflicts.

It is interesting to note that some homogeneous groups of workers who carry out jobs that are notoriously more demanding (such as teaching) were found to have "optimal" exposure levels, i.e. with no criticalities due to work-related stress. This can be explained by the fact that the work sheet does not assess the commitment and effort required to perform an activity, but whether the working conditions are sustainable without generating potential health impacts.

These characteristics are even more evident when analyzing the radar graphs obtained with the exposure assessment.

The first example (Figure 8.26) refers to the hospital kitchen described in the previous paragraph and compares it with the kitchen of a small nursery school. While the first setting is critical due to the high workload and low decision-making power, the second is optimal, and the greatest criticality lies in users with demands that are difficult to manage. Though both activities involve the preparation and distribution of food, the organizational approach, size of the facility and interpersonal relations among the workers differ considerably.

The radar graph is also very useful for deciding whether and which corrective actions are needed.

Another example concerns the homogeneous group of pediatric nurses (Figure 8.27); the final radar graph clearly shows that the average risk condition is mainly due to the workload, contact with human suffering and low decision-making power. On the other hand, the available tools and the working environment appear to be supportive. Corrective actions can thus focus on the three most challenging areas and the best solution would be to lower the workload. It is a well-known fact that rearranging workloads is not always feasible, so an alternative would be to find solutions that impact the other two sources of stress: increase decision-making power, increase staffing levels to compensate for the workload, or identify better forms of contact with users (patients), thus exposing staff to less human suffering.

The graph obtained from applying the work sheet to primary school teachers (Figure 8.28) shows that "optimal" exposure is determined by the characteristics of the occupation, that is, contact with users (pupils) sometimes with some difficulties and the workload, however, considerable decision-making power and the absence of other criticalities ensure excellent results in terms of exposure. In this case, the employer should make every effort to retain these working conditions.

As highlighted above, this result is obtained because the work sheet does not assess the commitment and effort required to perform a given activity, but rather the adequacy of the working conditions.

The result was different for a group of back-office bank employees (Figure 8.29). As can be seen, the exposure level is "acceptable", and the main criticality is the workload. In this case, corrective measures should focus mainly on the workload and on identifying ways to lighten it.

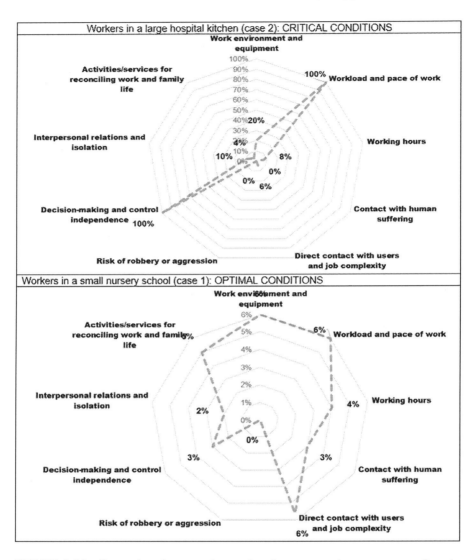

FIGURE 8.26 Comparison between the results of a pre-mapping assessment of work-related stress risk in two different homogeneous groups of kitchen workers in a large hospital and a small nursery school.

It is worth comparing this with the results for a homogeneous group of employees in a hospital outpatient clinic whose job involves booking clinical exams: the working conditions of these employees are critical due to their work-load, direct contact (sometimes tense) with the public and difficult interpersonal relations.

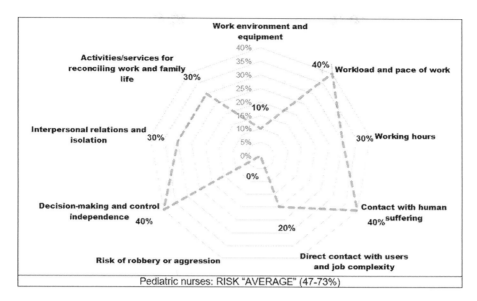

FIGURE 8.27   Results of a pre-mapping assessment of work-related stress risk in a homogeneous group of nurses in a small pediatric ward.

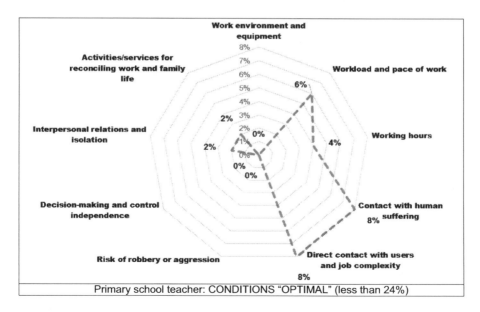

FIGURE 8.28   Results of a pre-mapping assessment of work-related stress risk in a homogeneous group of primary school teachers.

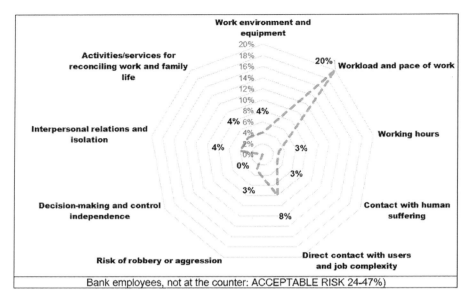

FIGURE 8.29 Results of a pre-mapping assessment of work-related stress risk in a homogeneous group of back-office bank staff.

8.10 CONCLUSIONS

The work sheet for assessing work-related stress, suitably included in the broader context of the ERGOCHECK software, is able to carry out both the pre-mapping of work-related stress risk in full compliance with European and Italian regulations, and also the actual preliminary risk assessment, for the same homogeneous group of workers for whom other risks have been mapped.

The work-related stress assessment work sheet does not claim to provide an extremely detailed risk analysis, or even to establish the level of job satisfaction of workers, but it is an excellent starting point for thinking about the risk of work-related stress in relation to the organizational and environmental setting within which the homogeneous group of workers perform their tasks.

As also shown by the final examples, an efficient organizational analysis and the effective collection of information from the workers and the employer (properly entered into the software provided by a trained and experienced operator) will accurately and quickly lead to a preliminary assessment of the risk associated with work-related stress, and to identifying the most appropriate and effective corrective and compensatory actions, based on the most critical psychosocial factors, thanks to this simple and intuitive approach.

The work sheet also lends itself to the compulsory education and training of Workers' Safety Representatives and members of homogeneous groups of workers, and the managers and supervisors in charge of implementing, supporting and facilitating preventive measures (Figure 8.30).

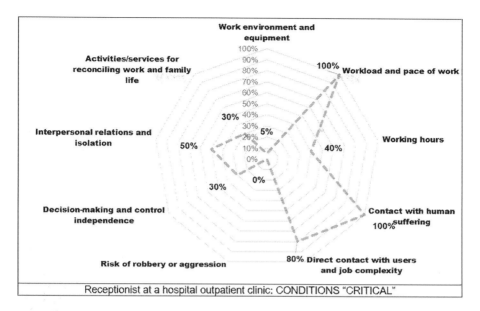

FIGURE 8.30 Results of a pre-mapping assessment of work-related stress risk in a homogeneous group of hospital outpatient clinic receptionists who schedule appointments.

9 Summary of Pre-mapping Evaluations by Homogeneous Group and Manufacturing Unit

Daniela Colombini and Enrico Occhipinti
Ergonomics of Posture and Movements
International Ergonomics School (EPM-IES)

CONTENTS

9.1   ERGOCHECK SUMMARIES BY HOMOGENEOUS GROUP

The results of the pre-mapping exercises carried out via *key enters/questions* and *quick assessments* can also be summarized graphically to more comprehensively define the "ERGOCHECK" objectives and corrective action priorities.

The summary is generated "automatically" in the last section of the spreadsheet.

The first section summarizes the evaluations of the various aspects relating to biomechanical overload (Figure 9.1). This section takes the evaluations carried out with the *quick assessment* process for repetitive movements, manual load handling (i.e. lifting, carrying and pulling/pushing) and for whole body postures (i.e. trunk and lower limbs). Specific percentages (from 0% to 100%) indicate the priority level for each of the aspects examined. Consequently, each aspect is rated, in the software designed to help in calculating the final exposure indices (**ERGOepmERGOCHECKpremapGLOBeng**), with colors indicating whether the issue is of negligible importance (green), somewhat significant (yellow), more important (red) extremely important or critical (purple).

Generally speaking, percentages of up to 30% are marked green, from 30% to 50% yellow, from 51% to 80% red and above 80% purple (absolute priority and/or critical).

The priority level for the manual handling of loads is expressed by combining additional elements with the actual overload elements which were instead listed separately in the summary of the specific work sheet.

113

For greater visual clarity no colors are depicted in Figure 9.1 but the levels are indicated by the percentages shown in the example.

The following summary covers all other risk factors or aspects examined (Figure 9.2). It is based on *key questions* or *quick assessments* for pollutants, biological agents and stress. The classification based on percentage priorities and colors is similar to that described for biomechanical overload.

B	CHECK / IDENTIFICATION OF PRIORITIES FOR BIOMECHANICAL OVERLOAD		
B1	BIOMECHANICAL OVERLOAD OF UPPER LIMBS IN REPETITIVE TASKS	Present	100%
B2	BIOMECHANICAL OVERLOAD - MANUAL LOAD LIFTING AND ADDITIONAL ENVIROMENTAL RISK FACTORS	Present	100%
B3	BIOMECHANICAL OVERLOAD - MANUAL LOAD CARRYING	Present	100%
B4	BIOMECHANICAL OVERLOAD - MANUAL PULLING AND PUSHING AND ADDITIONAL ENVIROMENTAL RISK FACTORS	Present	65%
B5	BIOMECHANICAL OVERLOAD - AWKWARD POSTURES OF SPINE AND LOWER LIMBS	Present	60%

FIGURE 9.1 Final summary of evaluations of various aspects relating to biomechanical overload (example of completed work sheet).

	CHECK / IDENTIFICATION OF PRIORITIES FOR OTHER WORKING CONDITIONS	
C	INDOOR LIGHTING PROBLEMS	0%
D	OUTDOOR WORK-RELATED PROBLEMS - UV RADIATION	25%
E	NOISE	75%
F	MICROCLIMATE PROBLEMS	50%
G	PROBLEMS ARISING FROM EQUIPMENT USE	100%
H	PROBLEMS RELATED TO VIBRATIONS	0%
I	MACHINERY-RELATED PROBLEMS	
J	ISSUES RELATED TO POLLUTANTS	100%
K	ISSUES RELATED TO BIOLOGICAL POLLUTANTS	0%
L	STRESS - ORGANIZATION	0%

FIGURE 9.2 Final summary of evaluations of other relevant factors or aspects (example of completed work sheet).

At the bottom of the summary section, a histogram (one for each factor examined) summarizes the level of priority and attention for all the factors examined (Figure 9.3). This, in fact, constitutes the actual "risk factor profile" for the homogeneous group and relevant processes included in the analysis.

Lastly, a string of values has been prepared in the Excel summary sheet (Figure 9.4); besides being the basis for the graph in Figure 9.3, these values can be applied to a different pre-mapping assessment of numerous homogeneous groups, as will be seen in Section 9.2.

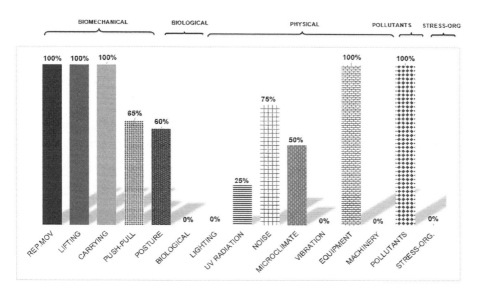

FIGURE 9.3 Graph summarizing pre-evaluation of all factors or aspects considered (example of completed work sheet).

REP.MOV	LIFTING	CARRYING	PUSH-PULL	POSTURE	BIOLOGICAL	LIGHTING	UV RADIATION	NOISE	MICROCLIMATE	VIBRATION	EQUIPMENT	MACHINERY	POLLUTANTS	STRESS-ORG.
100%	100%	100%	65%	60%	0%	0%	25%	75%	50%	0%	100%	0%	100%	0%

FIGURE 9.4 Horizontal list of pre-evaluation percentages for all factors or aspects considered (example of completed work sheet) for generating the graph presented in Figure 9.3 and for exporting to other spreadsheets.

9.2   SUMMARIES BY MANUFACTURING UNIT (AREA, DEPARTMENT, COMPANY): MAP OF COLLECTIVE RESULTS

When a company or manufacturing unit includes multiple homogeneous groups and therefore ERGOCHECK is used to produce many pre-mapping files, all the results need to be pooled in order to benefit from the outcome of a collective evaluation. In fact, it is not only useful but necessary to generate summaries for each manufacturing unit, be it a department, an area or even an entire company, if it is small. This is defined as a map of collective results.

Since it is impossible to "manually" manage the large amount of data involved, a specific Excel spreadsheet has been created (**ERGOepmERGOCHECKmapENG**), which will be presented in this chapter with an example application.

Figure 9.5 shows the header of the mapping software: this is where the data for the company in which the study has been carried out must first be entered. If it is a large company, it is possible to indicate only a single department or area.

The names of the homogeneous groups identified in a given area are first reported on the left-hand side of the first section of the Excel spreadsheet: the name of the area (department or other unit where the homogeneous groups operate) must be indicated in the appropriate box above the table in Figure 9.6. For each group (one per line), the following information must be entered:

- Net working hours;
- Number of breaks (based on data found in the ERGOCHECK REPETITIVE MOVEMENTS work sheet);
- Number of employees by gender (based on data found in the ERGOCHECK GENERAL work sheet), name of the homogeneous group and, if the work is rotated among workstations (as on an assembly line), name of the workstations.

The table in Figure 9.7 shows an example where, for each risk factor indicated and for each homogeneous group (horizontal line), the ERGOCHECK results are fully reported and appear in the final summary. To facilitate completing this final section

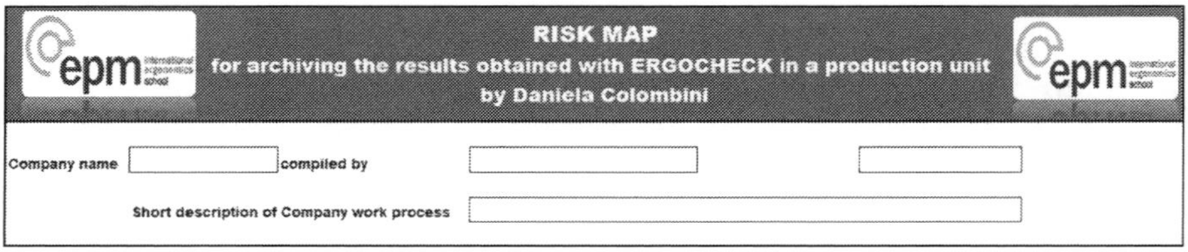

FIGURE 9.5   Risk map for filing the data obtained using ERGOCHECK: company data.

Net Duration of Repetitive Task	Breaks number in a representitive shift	MALE number in homogeneous group	FEMALE number in homogeneous group	Homogeneous group acronym	DATA REGARDING THE HOMOGENEOUS GROUPS PRESENT IN COMPANY: DEFINITION AND RISKS PROPORTIONAL DURATIONS						
					HOMOGENEOUS GROUP DEFINITION	Workstations worked by the homogeneous group					
440	3	4	3	G1	AAA						
440	2	5	10	G2	BBB						
440	2	2	6	G3	CCC						
440	3	10	4	G4	DDD						
440	5	1,0	5	G4	EEE						
440	2	10	1	G5	FFF						
440	1	5	1	G6	GGG						
440	2	2,0	8	G7	HHH						
440	3	1,0	5	G8	IIII						
440	3	2,0	2	G9	LLL						
180		6,0		G10	MMM						
180			10	G11	NNN						
440				G12							
440				G13							
440				G14							

FIGURE 9.6 ERGOCHECK collective map: first section with description of preliminary data characterizing the various homogeneous groups.

of ERGOCHECK, there is a "data strip" indicating the level, in percentage terms, of each risk factor (Figure 9.4, Section 9.1): the percentage lines can simply be copied from ERGOCHECK directly to the "data strips", thus created in the mapping (copy using the "paste values" button).

Even at first glance, the table indicates exposure levels to the various risk factors, for all the homogeneous groups working in the area under examination (software indicates exposure both as a percentage and as a color, from low to high (codes green, yellow, red and purple).

HOMOGENEOUS GROUP DEFINITION	REP MOV	LIFTING	CARRYING	PUSH-PULL	POSTURE	BIOLOGIC	LIGHTING	UV RADIATION	NOISE	MICROCLIMATE	VIBRATION	EQUIPMENT	MACHINERY	POLLUTANTS	STRESS-ORGAN	TOTAL	female	male
AAA	85%	50%	20%	33%	75%	65%	25%		24%	100%	65%	93%	13%	25%	43%	7	3	4
BBB	80%		50%	50%	35%		50%	50%	50%	20%	45%	50%	50%	45%	80%	15	10	5
CCC	50%			40%			20%		35%	50%		35%		50%	50%	8	6	2
DDD	25%	80%	40%	40%	75%		20%		40%		25%	25%	40%		20%	14	4	10
EEE	25%	30%			35%		35%			25%					30%	6	5	1
FFF								40%	45%	45%		45%				11	1	10
GGG			40%	40%	40%		40%									6	1	5
HHH	35%										35%	35%				10	8	2
IIII	23%						20%				20%					6	5	1
LLL	80%	40%	80%	80%	80%	80%	80%	80%	80%		80%		80%	80%		4	2	2
MMM	25%															6	0	6
NNN					35%					50%					80%	10	10	0
																0	0	0
																0	0	0
	49%	50%	46%	49%	57%	55%	38%	46%	46%	45%	49%	48%	46%	50%	51%	103	55	48

(Column header note: the "DATA REGARDING THE HOMOGENEOUS GROUPS PRESENT IN COMPANY: DEFINITION AND RISKS PROPORTIONAL DURATIONS" label heads the HOMOGENEOUS GROUP DEFINITION column.)

FIGURE 9.7 ERGOCHECK collective map: second section with data for each risk factor taken into consideration.

The same table also shows the number of workers exposed, per homogeneous group and as a total for the area, broken down by gender. The data entered in the previous section (Figure 9.7) is then processed and depicted in the following tables. Intervention priorities with respect to the different risk factors considered are immediately apparent thanks to the creation of three tables, each one extrapolating the risk factors causing similar discomfort levels and consequently with different intervention priorities, as follows:

- Mapping of urgent interventions, code purple (Figure 9.8);
- Mapping of medium-**term** interventions, code red (Figure 9.9);
- Mapping of non-urgent interventions, code yellow (Figure 9.10).

For each map, there is a comparison between the homogeneous groups present in the area, which risk factors associated with worker discomfort are to be investigated subsequently, and with which priority. The number of exposed workers per group and per risk factor are also indicated.

The last table (Figure 9.11) summarizes only the list of homogeneous groups for which there are:

- Only code yellow and/or code green results (for all risk factors);
- Only code green results (for all risk factors).

HOMOGENEOUS GROUPS THAT NEED AN URGENT RE-DESIGN INTERVENTION	REP MOV	LIFTING	CARRYING	PUSH-PULL	POSTURE	BIOLOGIC	LIGHTING	UV RADIATION	NOISE	MICROCLIMATE	VIBRATION	ATTREZZI	EQUIPMENT	POLLUTANTS	STRESS-ORGAN	female	male
AAA	85%									100%		93%				3	4
BBB	80%														80%	10	5
DDD		80%														4	10
LLL	80%		80%	80%	80%	80%	80%	80%	80%		80%		80%	80%		2	2
NNN															80%	10	0
0																0	0
0																0	0
0																0	0
	82%	80%	80%	80%	80%	80%	80%	80%	80%	100%	80%	93%	80%	80%	80%	29	21
NO. EXPOSED WORKERS	26	14	4	4	4	4	4	4	4	7	4	7	4	4	25	53%	44%

FIGURE 9.8 ERGOCHECK collective map. Results: map depicting workplace discomfort requiring URGENT INTERVENTION.

HOMOGENEOUS GROUPS THAT NEED A MEDIUM-TIME RE-DESIGN INTERVENTION	REP MOV	LIFTING	CARRYING	PUSH-PULL	POSTURE	BIOLOGIC	LIGHTING	UV RADIATION	NOISE	MICROCLIMATE	VIBRATION	ATTREZZI	EQUIPMENT	POLLUTANTS	STRESS-ORGAN	female	male
AAA		50%			75%	65%					65%					3	4
BBB			50%	50%			50%	50%	50%			50%	50%			10	5
CCC	60%									60%				50%	50%	6	2
DDD				75%												4	10
NNN										50%						10	0
0																0	0
0																0	0
0																0	0
	60%	50%	50%	50%	75%	65%	50%	50%	50%	50%	65%	50%	50%	50%	50%	33	21
NO. EXPOSED WORKER	8	7	15	15	21	7	15	15	15	18	7	15	15	8	8	60%	44%

FIGURE 9.9 ERGOCHECK collective map. Results: map depicting workplace discomfort requiring MEDIUM-TERM INTERVENTION.

HOMOGENEOUS GROUPS THAT DO NOT REQUIRE A SHORT-TIME RE-DESIGN INTERVENTION	REP. MOV	LIFTING	CARRYING	PUSH-PULL	POSTURE	BIOLOGIC	LIGHTING	UV RADIATION	NOISE	MICROCLIMATE	VIBRATION	ATTREZZI	EQUIPMENT	POLLUTANTS	STRESS-ORGAN.	female	male
AAA				33%											43%	3	4
BBB					35%						45%			45%		10	5
CCC			40%	40%	40%				35%			35%				6	2
DDD			40%	40%					40%				40%			4	10
EEE					35%		35%						45%			5	1
FFF								40%	45%	45%						0	0
GGG			40%	40%		40%		40%								1	5
HHH	35%										35%	35%				8	2
LLL		40%														2	2
NNN						35%										10	0
0																0	0
0																0	0
0																0	0
%	35%		46%	49%	49%		38%	46%	46%	45%	49%	48%	46%		43%	49 / 89%	31 / 65%
NO. EXPOSED WORKER	10	4	20	27	29	16	6	17	33	11	25	18	25	15	7		

FIGURE 9.10 ERGOCHECK collective map. Results: map depicting workplace discomfort NOT REQUIRING INTERVENTION.

HOMOGENEOUS GROUPS with results ONLY in RISK AREA YELLOW / GREEN	female	male	HOMOGENEOUS GROUPS with results ONLY in RISK AREA GREEN	female	male
EEE	5	1			
FFF	1	10			
GGG	1	5			
HHH	8	2			
IIII	5	1	IIII	5	1
MMM	0	6	MMM	0	6
	20	**25**		**5**	**7**
	36%	**52%**		**9%**	**15%**

FIGURE 9.11 ERGOCHECK collective map. Results: list of homogeneous groups with working conditions defined with different gray colors in function of the risk level: high, medium, low, absent.

The software then generates the levels of discomfort (again in percentages), this time for each risk factor and for all the homogeneous groups in the area under examination, for the total number of workers, and for both genders. The data is depicted in pie graphs with slices of different colors and sizes depending on the level of severity (from the lowest level, code green, to yellow, red and lastly purple) and quantitative presence (Figures 9.12a–e).

In conclusion, this is yet another simple tool for dealing quickly and easily with the critically important management of the results collected, in this specific instance, using the ERGOCHECK software.

It goes without saying that if the data is limited to only a few homogeneous groups working in a small business, this additional step might be unnecessary. But if there are many homogeneous groups working in a variety of places (areas, departments, etc.), in order to efficiently plan the next interventions (i.e. actual, more detailed, risk assessment or corrective measures in critical situations), a collective view of the results would be indispensable, albeit rather complex.

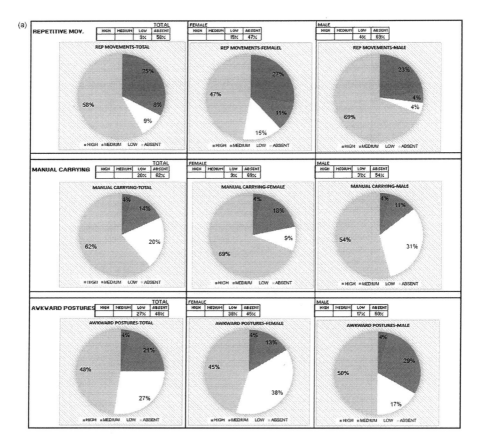

FIGURE 9.12 (a) ERGOCHECK collective map. Results: distribution of discomfort levels (in percentages) for each risk factor and for all the homogeneous groups working in the area under examination: REPETITIVE MOVEMENTS, MANUAL CARRYING, AWKWARD POSTURES. (b) ERGOCHECK collective map. Results: distribution of discomfort levels (in percentages) for each risk factor and for all the homogeneous groups working in the area under examination: MANUAL LIFTING, PUSHING AND PULLING, LIGHTING. (c) ERGOCHECK collective map. Results: distribution of discomfort levels (in percentages) for each risk factor and for all the homogeneous groups working in the area under examination: UV RADIATION, MICROCLIMATE, NOISE. (d) ERGOCHECK collective map. Results: distribution of discomfort levels (in percentages) for each risk factor and for all the homogeneous groups working in the area under examination: VIBRATIONS, EQUIPMENT, MACHINERY. (e) ERGOCHECK collective map. Results: distribution of discomfort levels (in percentages) for each risk factor and for all the homogeneous groups working in the area under examination: BIOLOGICAL POLLUTANTS, CHEMICAL POLLUTANTS AND PARTICULATES, STRESS-ORGANIZATION.

(Continued)

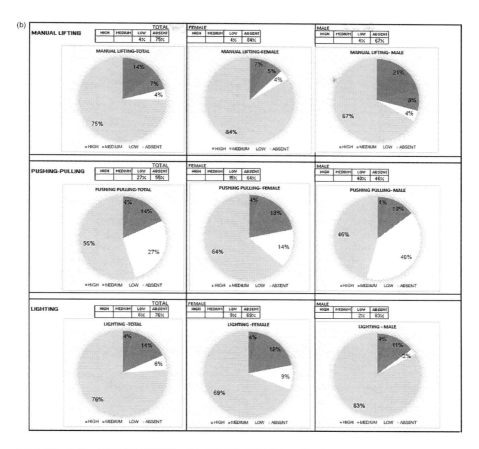

FIGURE 9.12 (CONTINUED) (a) ERGOCHECK collective map. Results: distribution of discomfort levels (in percentages) for each risk factor and for all the homogeneous groups working in the area under examination: REPETITIVE MOVEMENTS, MANUAL CARRYING, AWKWARD POSTURES. (b) ERGOCHECK collective map. Results: distribution of discomfort levels (in percentages) for each risk factor and for all the homogeneous groups working in the area under examination: MANUAL LIFTING, PUSHING AND PULLING, LIGHTING. (c) ERGOCHECK collective map. Results: distribution of discomfort levels (in percentages) for each risk factor and for all the homogeneous groups working in the area under examination: UV RADIATION, MICROCLIMATE, NOISE. (d) ERGOCHECK collective map. Results: distribution of discomfort levels (in percentages) for each risk factor and for all the homogeneous groups working in the area under examination: VIBRATIONS, EQUIPMENT, MACHINERY. (e) ERGOCHECK collective map. Results: distribution of discomfort levels (in percentages) for each risk factor and for all the homogeneous groups working in the area under examination: BIOLOGICAL POLLUTANTS, CHEMICAL POLLUTANTS AND PARTICULATES, STRESS-ORGANIZATION.

(Continued)

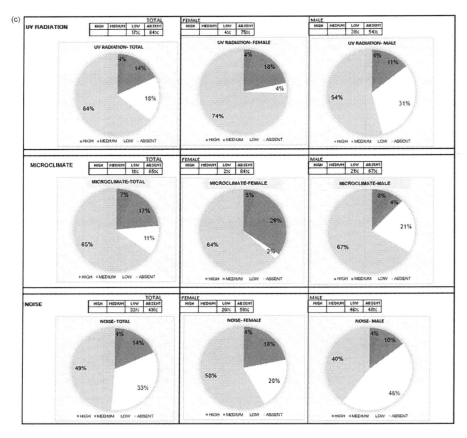

FIGURE 9.12 (CONTINUED) (a) ERGOCHECK collective map. Results: distribution of discomfort levels (in percentages) for each risk factor and for all the homogeneous groups working in the area under examination: REPETITIVE MOVEMENTS, MANUAL CARRYING, AWKWARD POSTURES. (b) ERGOCHECK collective map. Results: distribution of discomfort levels (in percentages) for each risk factor and for all the homogeneous groups working in the area under examination: MANUAL LIFTING, PUSHING AND PULLING, LIGHTING. (c) ERGOCHECK collective map. Results: distribution of discomfort levels (in percentages) for each risk factor and for all the homogeneous groups working in the area under examination: UV RADIATION, MICROCLIMATE, NOISE. (d) ERGOCHECK collective map. Results: distribution of discomfort levels (in percentages) for each risk factor and for all the homogeneous groups working in the area under examination: VIBRATIONS, EQUIPMENT, MACHINERY. (e) ERGOCHECK collective map. Results: distribution of discomfort levels (in percentages) for each risk factor and for all the homogeneous groups working in the area under examination: BIOLOGICAL POLLUTANTS, CHEMICAL POLLUTANTS AND PARTICULATES, STRESS-ORGANIZATION.

(Continued)

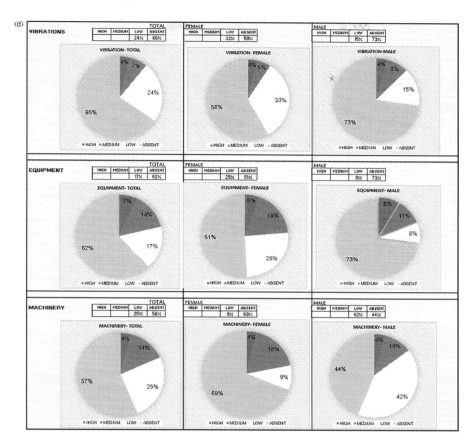

FIGURE 9.12 (CONTINUED) (a) ERGOCHECK collective map. Results: distribution of discomfort levels (in percentages) for each risk factor and for all the homogeneous groups working in the area under examination: REPETITIVE MOVEMENTS, MANUAL CARRYING, AWKWARD POSTURES. (b) ERGOCHECK collective map. Results: distribution of discomfort levels (in percentages) for each risk factor and for all the homogeneous groups working in the area under examination: MANUAL LIFTING, PUSHING AND PULLING, LIGHTING. (c) ERGOCHECK collective map. Results: distribution of discomfort levels (in percentages) for each risk factor and for all the homogeneous groups working in the area under examination: UV RADIATION, MICROCLIMATE, NOISE. (d) ERGOCHECK collective map. Results: distribution of discomfort levels (in percentages) for each risk factor and for all the homogeneous groups working in the area under examination: VIBRATIONS, EQUIPMENT, MACHINERY. (e) ERGOCHECK collective map. Results: distribution of discomfort levels (in percentages) for each risk factor and for all the homogeneous groups working in the area under examination: BIOLOGICAL POLLUTANTS, CHEMICAL POLLUTANTS AND PARTICULATES, STRESS-ORGANIZATION.

(Continued)

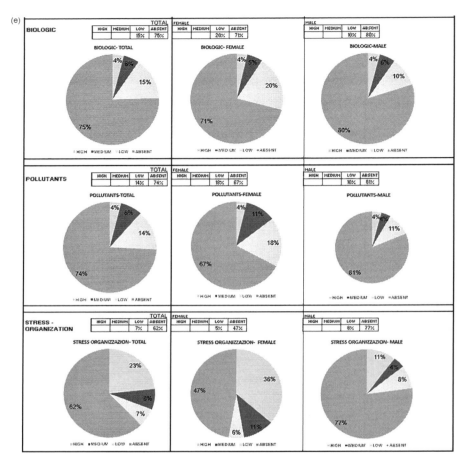

FIGURE 9.12 (CONTINUED) (a) ERGOCHECK collective map. Results: distribution of discomfort levels (in percentages) for each risk factor and for all the homogeneous groups working in the area under examination: REPETITIVE MOVEMENTS, MANUAL CARRYING, AWKWARD POSTURES. (b) ERGOCHECK collective map. Results: distribution of discomfort levels (in percentages) for each risk factor and for all the homogeneous groups working in the area under examination: MANUAL LIFTING, PUSHING AND PULLING, LIGHTING. (c) ERGOCHECK collective map. Results: distribution of discomfort levels (in percentages) for each risk factor and for all the homogeneous groups working in the area under examination: UV RADIATION, MICROCLIMATE, NOISE. (d) ERGOCHECK collective map. Results: distribution of discomfort levels (in percentages) for each risk factor and for all the homogeneous groups working in the area under examination: VIBRATIONS, EQUIPMENT, MACHINERY. (e) ERGOCHECK collective map. Results: distribution of discomfort levels (in percentages) for each risk factor and for all the homogeneous groups working in the area under examination: BIOLOGICAL POLLUTANTS, CHEMICAL POLLUTANTS AND PARTICULATES, STRESS-ORGANIZATION.

10 Examples of ERGOCHECK Spreadsheets[1]

Daniela Colombini and Enrico Occhipinti
Ergonomics of Posture and Movements
International Ergonomics School (EPM-IES)

CONTENTS

10.1 THE EXAMPLE

The example is that of a group of stone cutters who work on serpentine, a stone that can be found in the Valtellina region of northern Italy that is used as slate for roofing and building façades. The homogeneous group is comprised of four workers, who perform the same tasks during the shift, in a "workshop" (a simple and old-fashioned) to which blocks of stone (weighing from 25 to 50 kg) coming from a quarry are delivered.

They do not work down a mine.

The large blocks are transported to the workshop by hand pallet truck, where they are first cut into smaller slabs weighing between 10 and 25 kg (Figure 10.1) using hand tools (in particular mallets and chisels), which are then generally moved by hand. These slabs are split into precious stone slates (serpentine is in fact a very expensive material) each weighing approximately 3–4 kg (Figure 10.2). The stone slabs must be split along the natural bedding planes of the stone: this requires great skill and experience. The stone contains silica: in the quarry asbestos veins may be

---

[1] This chapter will illustrate how to complete the ERGOCHECK spreadsheets, using a concrete example.

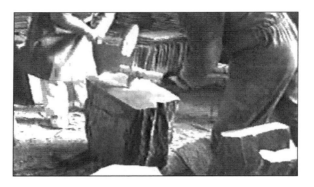

FIGURE 10.1   Splitting blocks of serpentine.

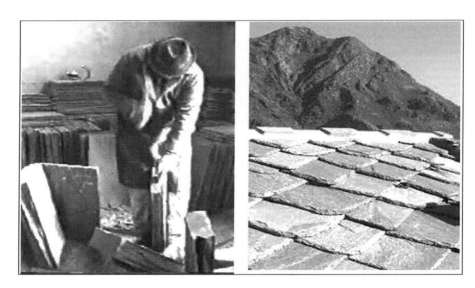

FIGURE 10.2   Cutting slabs of serpentine.

found close to the serpentine. The work is repetitive and high-risk, given the presence of peak force. Manually lifted loads can exceed 25 kg. There are also problems associated with the pulling and pushing of hand pallet trucks due to the conditions of the soil outside the workshop. Noise and the microclimate are generally also a problem; the tools are obsolete and could cause accidents or injuries. There is silica dust (and possibly also asbestos), although sledgehammers are used to cut the stone and not grinders. The workshop has no dust aspirators.

In this example, a homogeneous group of workers performs several tasks, from transporting stone with hand pallet trucks, to carrying them manually, cutting the stone and placing it in the storage area. However, just one pre-mapping work sheet must be compiled: the questionnaire is not for the entire company or for a single task but should be used to describe a complete task performed by a specific homogeneous group of workers.

10.2   COMPLETING THE ERGOCHECK WORK SHEETS

10.2.1   PART 1: FIRST SECTION ON THE MAIN CAUSES
OF DISCOMFORT AND DANGER

The first work sheet begins with the data concerning the company and the homogeneous group under examination (Figure 10.3)

Next, the *key enters for* the various conditions of *biomechanical overload* are checked.

In the example, all the conditions for biomechanical overload are positive (Figures 10.4 and 10.5); therefore, the respective *quick assessments* will need to be completed.

Next, physical risk factors are examined via *key questions*.

Lighting: In the example, the workers report that general and localized lighting are both satisfactory; the materials are not shiny and do not cause glare (Figure 10.6).

A	COMPANY DATA AND TASKS ANALYZED		
Company name	AAAA	Process	CCCC
Industry	BBBB	No. of employees	Males 4,0 / Females
Address	XXXX		
Other details	YYYY		
Short description of process	The 4 workers operate within a "laboratory" (modest and antiquated). On the external square, blocks of stone (from 25 to 50 kg) extracted from the quarry are unloaded from other workers. With manual pallet trucks, these blocks are transported inside the laboratory where, with manual tools (in particular bat and chisels), they are first divided into smaller pieces, weighing from 10 to 25 kg, which are then generally handled manually. From these pieces, using bat and smal chisels, stone slabs are obtained, with an indicative weight of 3-4 kg. each.		

FIGURE 10.3   ERGOCHECK: data identifying and company and homogeneous group.

B1	BIOMECHANICAL OVERLOAD OF UPPER LIMBS IN REPETITIVE TASKS	
	PRESENCE OF REPETITIVE TASKS: The task is organized in cycles, regardless of their duration, or the task is characterized by similar working gestures for over 50% of the time. The term "repetitive" does not mean risk is present.	YES x / NO Go directly to work sheet REPETITIVE-MOV
B2	BIOMECHANICAL OVERLOAD FROM MANUAL HANDLING - LIFTING	
	PRESENCE OF OBJECTS WEIGHING 3 KG OR MORE TO BE MANUALLY LIFTED (if the loads are lighter, there is no need to continue the investigation)	YES x / NO Go directly to work sheet MANUAL HANDLING
B3	BIOMECHANICAL OVERLOAD FROM MANUAL HANDLING - CARRYING	
	PRESENCE OF OBJECTS WEIGHING 3 KG OR MORE TO BE MANUALLY CARRIED (if the loads are lighter, there is no need to continue the investigation).	YES x / NO Go directly to work sheet MANUAL HANDLING
B4	BIOMECHANICAL OVERLOAD FROM MANUAL PUSHING AND PULLING	
	IS THERE WHOLE-BODY PUSHING OR PULLING OF LOADS?	YES x / NO Go directly to work sheet MANUAL HANDLING

FIGURE 10.4   Key enters for biomechanical overload due to repetitive movements and manual load handling.

B5	BIOMECHANICAL OVERLOAD FROM AWKWARD POSTURES - TRUNK AND LOWER LIMBS		

	YES	x
Are there static or awkward working postures of the HEAD/NECK, TRUNK and/or UPPER AND LOWER LIMBS maintained for more than 4 seconds consecutively and repeated for a significant proportion of the working time?	**YES**	x
Generally speaking, **working postures are not awkward (INDICATE "NO")** when the subject: - is sitting with the back well supported, adequate leg room and can stand up (change position) at least every hour. - is standing with the trunk erect (no deep bending or twisting) but free to walk around or sit at least every hour (with the back well supported and adequate leg room).	**NO**	

i.e.		NO	YES
	HEAD/NECK (neck bent back/forward/sideways, twisted)		x
	TRUNK (trunk bent forward/sideways/, back bent with no support, twisted)		x
	UPPER LIMBS (hand(s) at or above head, elbow(s) at or above shoulder level, elbow/hand(s) behind the body, hand(s) turned with palms completely up or down, extreme elbow flexion-extension, wrist bent forward/backward/sideways)		
	LOWER LIMBS (squatting or kneeling) with position maintained for more than 4 seconds consecutively and repeated for a significant proportion of the working time		

Please, proceed to the sheet POSTURES for trunk
and lower limbs or to sheet REPETITIVE-MOV for
upper limbs

FIGURE 10.5   Key enters for biomechanical overload due to awkward postures.

C	KEY-QUESTIONS FOR IDENTIFYING INDOOR LIGHTING PROBLEMS		
GENERAL LIGHTING: ASSESSMENT OF VISUAL EFFORT AT WORK			
SUFFICIENT			x
POOR :	FOR A FEW HOURS A DAY		
	ALL DAY		
EXCESSIVE:	FOR A FEW HOURS A DAY		
	ALL DAY		
ARTIFICIAL LIGHTING: NEEDED BUT UNAVAILABLE			
LOCALIZED LIGHTING. ASSESSMENT OF VISUAL EFFORT AT WORK			
SUFFICIENT			x
POOR :	FOR A FEW HOURS A DAY		
	ALL DAY		
EXCESSIVE:	FOR A FEW HOURS A DAY		
	ALL DAY		
NEEDED BUT UNAVAILABLE			
BENCH OR TABLE TOPS	MATTE		
	BRIGHT AND SHINY		
SURFACES OF OBJECTS	MATTE		x
BEING PROCESSED	BRIGHT AND SHINY		

FIGURE 10.6   Key questions on lighting.

Exposure to UV radiation: In this work setting, the tasks are generally performed indoors and only occasionally (in summer) outdoors with exposure to direct sunlight. The possible answers were, therefore, "Occasional" or, more cautiously "Exposure for a significant proportion of the year"; the latter was checked. There is, of course, no welding (Figure 10.7).

D	**KEY-QUESTIONS FOR OUTDOOR WORK-RELATED PROBLEMS - UV**	
	Exposure to UV radiation and/or weather	
INDOOR WORK		
OCCASIONAL OUTDOOR WORK		
OUTDOOR WORK FOR A SIGNIFICANT PROPORTION OF THE YEAR (1/3)		x
OUTDOOR WORK FOR MORE THAN HALF OF THE YEAR (2/3)		
OUTDOOR WORK NEARLY ALL YEAR (3/3)		

FIGURE 10.7   Key questions on exposure to UV radiation.

Noise: Although the work does not normally require verbal communications with co-workers (or customers), the level of perceived noise is very high (hammering on stone) and such as to hinder dialog between people. The task does not require continuous verbal communications with co-workers (Figure 10.8).

Microclimate: Since the work is carried out in environments with inadequate heating and no air conditioning, it was reported as hot during summer and cold during winter (Figure 10.9).

E	**KEY-QUESTIONS FOR IDENTIFYING NOISE-RELATED HAZARDS**	
	Perceived noise level	
The task calls for verbal communications with CO-WORKERS		
THE NOISE DOES NOT BOTHER		
THE NOISE BOTHERS A LITTLE, BUT IT IS POSSIBLE TO TALK TO CO-WORKERS		
THE NOISE IS MADDENING, IT IS DIFFICULT TO TALK TO CO-WORKERS		
THE NOISE IS VERY LOUD, IT IS IMPOSSIBLE TO TALK TO CO-WORKERS		
The task does not call for any verbal communications with CO-WORKERS		
THE NOISE DOES NOT BOTHER		
THE NOISE BOTHERS A LITTLE, BUT IT IS POSSIBLE TO TALK TO CO-WORKERS		
THE NOISE IS MADDENING, IT IS DIFFICULT TO TALK TO CO-WORKERS		
THE NOISE IS VERY LOUD, IT IS IMPOSSIBLE TO TALK TO CO-WORKERS		x

FIGURE 10.8   Key questions on noise.

F	**KEY-QUESTIONS FOR MICROCLIMATE-RELATED PROBLEMS**	
	WORKING INDOORS WITH NO EXPOSURE TO THE WEATHER	
COMFORTABLE ALL YEAR		
IT IS HOT:	ONLY IN SUMMER	x
	ALL YEAR	
IT IS COLD:	ONLY IN WINTER	x
	ALL YEAR	
WORKING OUTDOORS WITH EXPOSURE TO THE WEATHER		
ONLY IN SUMMER		
ONLY IN WINTER		
ALL YEAR		

FIGURE 10.9   Key questions on microclimate.

Use of manual tools: In this case, multiple answers are possible and the more responses checked the problem with the highest priority. Here, many unfavorable conditions have been ticked, both by the workers and by the outside observer (Figure 10.10).

Vibrations: Figure 10.11 assesses the presence of hand-arm vibration (vibrating tools) and whole-body vibration (driving vehicles). In this case, the workers reported the occasional and sporadic use of pneumatic chisels for cutting down the large blocks that arrive from the quarry.

Use of machinery: The *key questions* are similar to those for manual tools.

The stone cutters do not use machinery; therefore, this work sheet was not completed.

The next step is to return to the *key enters* for pollutants (chemical, biological or particulate matter).

In the example, there is clearly high exposure to silica-rich dust rich with possible traces of asbestos (Figure 10.12). The pre-assessment will be completed with

G KEY-QUESTIONS FOR PROBLEMS ARISING FROM EQUIPMENT USE	
ADEQUATE AND WELL-MAINTAINED	
HEAVY	x
NOISY	x
REQUIRES STRENGTH	x
NOT WORKING WELL	
CUMBERSOME AND/OR HARD TO GRASP	
NOT FIT FOR SPECIFIC USE AND/OR TECHNOLOGICALLY BACKWARD	x
OVERHEATS EASILY	
REQUIRES EXCESSIVE ATTENTION	
MAY PRODUCE LESIONS (CUTS, SCRATCHES, BLISTERS, BURNS, ETC.)	x
BODY PARTS USED AS EQUIPMENT WITH CONSEQUENT LESIONS (CALLUSES, RASHES, CUTS, ETC.)	

FIGURE 10.10   Key questions on the use of tools.

H KEY-QUESTIONS FOR PROBLEMS RELATED TO VIBRATIONS	
NO EXPOSURE TO VIBRATIONS	
The task calls for the use of vibrating tools	
OCCASIONALLY	x
SCREWDRIVERS AT LEAST 1/3 OF THE TIME	
GRINDERS/CUTTERS/POLISHERS AT LEAST 1/3 OF THE TIME	
JACKHAMMERS AT LEAST 1/3 OF THE TIME	
The task involves driving	
OCCASIONALLY	
MOST OF THE TIME DRIVING CARS, MOTORCYCLES, VANS	
MOST OF THE TIME DRIVING TRUCKS, BUSES	
MOST OF THE TIME DRIVING TRACTORS, FARM VEHICLES, SCRAPERS, DIGGERS	

FIGURE 10.11   Key questions on exposure to vibration.

J	KEY-QUESTIONS FOR PROBLEMS ASSOCIATED WITH BIOLOGICAL OR OTHER POLLUTANTS		
		proceed to the sheet POLLUTANTS	
NO BIOLOGICAL OR OTHER POLLUTANTS PRESENT			
DUST: specify type		PRESENT	
	silica	SIGNIFICANT PRESENCE	X
FUMES: specify type		PRESENT	
		SIGNIFICANT PRESENCE	
UNPLEASANT ODORS: describe		PRESENT	
		SIGNIFICANT PRESENCE	
CHEMICALS: specify type		PRESENT	
		SIGNIFICANT PRESENCE	
BIOLOGICAL POLLUTANTS		PRESENT	
		SIGNIFICANT PRESENCE	

FIGURE 10.12 Key enters for the presence of chemical, physical or biological agents.

the appropriate *quick assessment* work sheet. There is no significant exposure to biological agents; therefore, the relevant *quick assessment* work sheet will be disregarded.

Lastly, it is worth noting that, with respect to the organizational aspects and stress, in this example, there is a daily shift of about 8 hours, with no set pace or pro-ductivity bonuses, and without any significant overtime; it did not appear necessary to investigate work-related stress (the four workers are in fact the "master craftsmen" and did not report any organizational problems or relationship issues). The relevant *quick assessment* work sheet was, therefore, disregarded.

10.2.2 PART 2: REPETITIVE MOVEMENTS OF THE UPPER LIMBS

As the *key enter* for repetitive movements was checked, the corresponding *quick assessment* work sheet needs to be completed.

In this case, the first section of the work sheet briefly describes the duration of the repetitive work and of breaks (Figure 10.13).

Summary of repetitive work net duration on a representative average day			
TOTAL shift average duration (in minutes)	480	Total repetitive working time (in minutes)	390

DESCRIPTION OF NON-REPETITIVE TASKS, THEIR DURATION AND TIMING OF BREAKS - TOTAL DURATION	
supply	
cleaning	30
other	30
Total duration of non-repetitive work per shift (in minutes)	60
Breaks (average) total duration per shift (in minutes): including meal break only if included in the shift	30
Number of breaks (including meal break) lasting at least 8 minutes	3

FIGURE 10.13 Quick assessment of repetitive movements: description of working hours and breaks.

The next sections are completed, as per ISO/TR 12295, which identify potentially acceptable or critical conditions (Figure 10.14).

In the example, the working conditions cannot be defined as acceptable because "NO" was answered to two items (movement time of the upper limbs and use of force) in the relevant section. Conversely, the conditions are "critical" because there is use of "peak force" (i.e. sledgehammers to reduce large blocks of stone) for more than 10% of the total working hours.

As the condition has been found to be critical, it is not necessary (the section does not appear in the software) to complete the more detailed work sheet for evaluating conditions found to be neither fully acceptable nor clearly critical.

At the bottom of the page, there is also a summary of the pre-assessment of repetitive movements, with an indication of the relative intervention priorities (Figure 10.15). In this specific example, the first intervention should consist in eliminating the use of peak force due to the use of sledgehammers.

ACCEPTABLE CONDITIONS				
*If all conditions are described and replies are all **YES**, the risk level is acceptable for repetitive work and it is not necessary to continue the risk evaluation.*				
Are one or both upper limbs used for less than 50% of the total duration of the repetitive task(s)?	No	X	Yes	
Are both elbows held below shoulder level almost 90% of the total duration of the repetitive task(s)?	No		Yes	X
Is moderate or no force required (perceived effort = max 3 or 4 on CR-10 Borg scale) by the operator for no more than 1 hour for the duration of the repetitive task(s) and are there no force peaks (perceived effort = 5 or more on CR-10 Borg scale)?	No	X	Yes	
Are there breaks (including meal breaks) lasting at least 8 min every 2 hours and is the repetitive task performed for less than 8 hours a day?	No		Yes	X
CRITICAL CONDITIONS				
*If at least one of the following conditions is present (**YES**), risk must be considered as CRITICAL and task re-design is URGENTLY REQUIRED.*				
Are technical actions performed with a single limb so fast that they cannot be counted by simple direct observation?	No	X	Yes	
Are one or both arms used to perform the task with elbow(s) at shoulder level for half or more than the total repetitive working time?	No	X	Yes	
Is a "pinch" grip (or any type of grasp using the finger tips) held for more than 80% of the repetitive working time?	No	X	Yes	
Is peak force applied (perceived effort = 5 or more on the CR-10 Borg scale) for 10% or more of the total repetitive working time?	No		Yes	X
Is there only one break (including meal break) in a shift of 6-8 hours, or does the total repetitive working time exceed 8 hours in the shift?	No	X	Yes	

FIGURE 10.14 Quick assessment of repetitive movements: examination of potentially "acceptable" and "critical" conditions.

BIOMECHANICAL OVERLOAD OF THE UPPER LIMBS IN REPETITIVE TASKS	
SUMMARY OF PRE-ASSESSMENT AND INTERVENTION PRIORITIES	A critical condition is present. The risk is surely high.
	Intervention is urgent.

FIGURE 10.15 Quick assessment of repetitive movements: summary of pre-assessment and indication of intervention priorities.

10.2.3 PART 3: MANUAL LOAD HANDLING

This work sheet provides for a *quick assessment* of the various aspects of manual load handling (lifting, carrying, pushing/pulling).

In the example, all these aspects were checked via the *key enters* in Part 1, and as such need to be further investigated in Part 3.

In accordance with ISO/TR 12295, first of all the "additional factors" for lifting and carrying are examined, some of which have been ticked in this example (Figure 10.16).

The next step is to check whether there are "critical" conditions for lifting: in this example, since loads weighing more than 25 kg are also lifted, conditions are "critical" (Figure 10.17). As a result, there is no point filling in the section on potentially "acceptable" conditions (which in any case would require loads to weigh less than 10 kg), or the section on conditions somewhere between "acceptable" and "critical" (generally, with loads weighing between 10 and 25 kg). If in doubt, however, it is advisable to complete all the sections relating to lifting.

The evaluation then goes on to examine manual carrying tasks (Figure 10.18).

Additional ORGANIZATIONAL AND ENVIROMENTAL risk factors				
Is the working environment unfavorable for manual lifting and carrying?				
Presence of extreme (low or high) temperatures	No	X	Yes	
Presence of slippery, uneven, unstable floors	No		Yes	X
Presence of insufficient space for lifting and carrying	No		Yes	X
Are objects unfavorable for manual lifting and carrying?				
The size of object reduces the operator's view and hinders movement	No	X	Yes	
The centre of gravity of the load is not stable (for example: liquids, items moving around inside the object)	No	X	Yes	
The object's shape/configuration features sharp edges, surfaces or protrusions	No		Yes	X
The contact surfaces are too cold or too hot	No	X	Yes	
Does the task with manual lifting or carrying last more than 8 hours a day?	No	X	Yes	

FIGURE 10.16 Quick assessment of manual lifting: additional factors for lifting and carrying.

CRITICAL CONDITIONS					
If only one of aforementioned conditions is present (YES), the risk is to be considered as high and the task must be immediately re-designed.					
Task lay-out and frequency					
VERTICAL LOCATION	The hand location at the beginning/end of the lift is higher than 175 cm or lower than 0 cm	No	X	Yes	
VERTICAL DISPLACEMENT	The vertical distance between the origin and the destination of the lifted object is more than 175cm	No	X	Yes	
HORIZONTAL DISTANCE	The horizontal distance between the body and load is greater than full arm reach	No	X	Yes	
ASYMMETRY	Extreme body twisting without moving the feet	No	X	Yes	
FREQUENCY	equal to or higher than 15 times/minute for SHORT DURATION (MAX 60 min)	No	X	Yes	
	equal to or higher than 12 times/minute for MEDIUM DURATION (MAX 120 min)	No	X	Yes	
	equal to or higher than 8 times/minute for LONG DURATION (OVER 120 min)	No	X	Yes	
Presence of loads exceeding the following limits					
men (18-45 years)	25 KG	No		Yes	X
women (18-45 years)	20 KG	No	X	Yes	
men (<18 or >45 years)	20 KG	No		Yes	X
women (<18 or >45 years)	15 KG	No	X	Yes	

FIGURE 10.17 Quick assessment of manual lifting: assessment of potentially critical conditions.

Conditions of manual load carrying					
REPRESENTATIVE DURATION OF CARRYiNG IN THE SHIFT (min.)	390,0	min			
No. of objects exceeding 3 KG carried in the shift	Weight of objects moved	Cumulative mass (KG)		Max Distance	4m - 10m
200,0	3,0	600,0			
60,0	14,0	840,0			
10,0	27,0	270,0	Loads weighted more than 25kg are present!		
		0,0			
Cumulative Mass (total load carried in the shift)		1710,0	Does not exceed the limit		
Estimated cumulative mass per hour		263,1	Does not exceed the limit		
Estimated cumulative mass per minute		4,4	It does not exceed the limit		
Are loads carried under unfavorable environmental conditions or lifted from/to low heights, e.g. below knee level or above shoulders?				No	Yes x

FIGURE 10.18   Quick assessment of manual carrying.

In this case, the first step is to enter the essential data relating to the time frame during which loads are carried (in minutes in the shift). Next, to calculate the total mass carried, the number and respective weight of the loads carried (and probably previously lifted) must be indicated. The modal range of the carrying distance also needs specifying. Lastly, it should be indicated whether the carrying takes place under favorable or unfavorable conditions.

In this example, since it is indicated that the workers carry (as well as lift) objects weighing over 25 kg (on average ten times per shift) the conditions are critical. If the conditions are not critical (loads weighing less than the reported limits), the software calculates the total mass carried and compares it with the limits set out in ISO 11228-1 (respectively, for 8 hours, 1 hour and 1 minute), over different carrying distances.

Lastly, manual pushing/pulling (hand pallet trucks in this case) also needs examining (*key enter* checked).

As mentioned above, the first information to be collected, using the Borg CR-10 scale, concerns the effort perceived by the workers in their pushing/pulling tasks. The next step is to verify the potential presence of additional factors that may affect the same tasks. In this case, the perceived effort was more or less moderate (3 on the Borg scale), with evidence of some additional factors (Figure 10.19).

IS THERE WHOLE-BODY PUSHING OR PULLING OF LOADS?			
IF PRESENT, SPECIFY THE BORG SCALE VALUE IN THE WHITE BOX BELOW			
Perceived effort (obtained by interviewing workers using the CR-10 Borg scale):		3,0 - moderate	
Additional organizational and enviromental risk factors to be considered			
Is the working environment unfavourable for pushing or pulling?			
Are floors slippery, unstable, uneven, upward or downward sloping or cracked/broken?	No	Yes	X
Are there restricted or obstructed paths?	No	Yes	X
Is the temperature of the working area high?	No X	Yes	
Are objects unfavorable for pushing or pulling?			
Does the object (or trolley, pallet, etc.) limit the view of the operator or hinder movement?	No X	Yes	
Is the object unstable?	No X	Yes	
Does the object (or trolley, pallet, etc.) have hazardous features, sharp surfaces, projections etc. that could injure the operator?	No X	Yes	
Are the wheels or casters worn, broken or not properly maintained?	No	Yes	X
Are the wheels or casters unsuitable for the working conditions?	No X	Yes	

FIGURE 10.19   Quick assessment of manual pushing and pulling: perceived effort and analysis of additional factors.

After that comes a section checking for the presence of potentially acceptable vs. critical conditions for pushing/pulling according to ISO/TR 12295 (Figure 10.20).

Given the preliminary determination of effort perceived as moderate, the condition will obviously not be fully acceptable. However, nor is it clearly critical. In reality, given the description provided, the situation sits half a way between the two extremes and with an average priority level in light of the results of the Borg scale survey.

Part 3 "Manual Load Handling" concludes with a summary of the evaluations and resulting priorities (Figure 10.21). It is worth noting that the "additional aspects" with regard to lifting/carrying and pushing/pulling, respectively, are summarized separately from the proper evaluation of biomechanical overload in the stricter sense.

ACCEPTABLE CONDITIONS				
If all conditions are met and replies are all YES, the risk level is acceptable for pushing-pulling tasks. However, additional factors must be checked (see above).				
Does the perceived effort (obtained by interviewing workers using the CR-10 Borg scale) show the presence during pushing-pulling task(s) of up to SLIGHT exertione (perceived effort - score 2 or less in Borg CR-10 scale)?	No	X	Yes	
Is the manual pushing and pulling work performed for up to 8 hours a day?	No		Yes	X
Is pushing-pulling force applied to the object between hip and mid-chest height?	No		Yes	X
Is the pushing-pulling work performed with an upright trunk (not twisted or bent)?	No		Yes	X
Are hands held within shoulder width and in front of the body?	No		Yes	X

CRITICAL CONDITIONS				
If even only one of these conditions is present (YES), the risk is to be considered as high and the task must be immediately re-designed.				
Does the perceived effort using the CR-10 Borg scale (obtained by interviewing the workers) show the presence of high peaks of force (perceived effort, with a score of 8 or more on the Borg CR-10 scale)?	No	X	Yes	
Is the pushing-pulling work performed with the trunk significantly bent or twisted?	No	X	Yes	
Is the pushing-pulling work performed in a jerky or uncontrolled manner?	No	X	Yes	
Are hands held either wider than shoulder width or not in front of the body?	No	X	Yes	
Hands are held higher than 150 cm or lower than 60 cm.	No	X	Yes	
Together with the pushing-pulling work is there also use of vertical force ("partial lifting")?	No	X	Yes	
Does the task(s) with manual pushing and pulling lasts more than 8 hours a day?	No	X	Yes	

FIGURE 10.20 Quick assessment of manual pushing and pulling: analysis of potentially "acceptable" and "critical" conditions.

Summary of quick assessment for manual load handling	
BIOMECHANICAL OVERLOAD FOR MANUAL LIFTING	
SUMMARY OF PRE-ASSESSMENT AND INTERVENTION PRIORITIES	A critical condition is present. The risk is surely high.
	Urgent intervention required.
BIOMECHANICAL OVERLOAD FOR MANUAL CARRYING	
SUMMARY OF PRE-ASSESSMENT AND INTERVENTION PRIORITIES	Risk assessment necessary.
	Urgent intervention required.
Summary of enviromental additional factors important for MMH	
	Presence of significative enviromental problems
BIOMECHANICAL OVERLOAD FOR PUSHING and PULLING	
SUMMARY OF PRE-ASSESSMENT AND INTERVENTION PRIORITIES	Risk assessment necessary.
	Risk assessment advisable as soon as possible
Summary of additional enviromental factors THAT ARE SIGNIFICANT for PUSHING and PULLING	
	Presence of significative enviromental problems

FIGURE 10.21 Final summary of quick assessment of various aspects regarding manual load handling.

10.2.4 Part 4: Postures of the Trunk and Lower Limbs

The first section concerns postures of the trunk (Figure 10.22).

In the example, these are standing postures and for a certain percentage of the working hours (30%) involve keeping the back straight, while most of the time (60%) the back is slightly bent. The remaining 10% of the time is spent with the back bending forward deeply.

It is worth noting that the description of postures (in this case of the trunk) requires indicating the proportion of time spent in the various postures indicated in the table. Even if the percentages may be approximate (no unnecessary details are called for), in any case the total sum must be equal to 100% (i.e. the entire work shift).

The postures of the lower limbs are described next (Figure 10.23).

Trunk posture Standing or squatting (not seated)		
Nearly always upright		30%
Frequent moderate bending		60%
Frequent twisting		
Frequent deep bending		10%
Seated		
Leaning on the back rest		
Upright without backrest		
Mostly bending forward		
Frequent twisting of trunk		
Note:	Described time of trunk posture:	100%

FIGURE 10.22 Quick assessment of postures of the trunk.

Lower limb postures Standing or squatting (not seated)		
Standing and able to walk around		50%
Standing in a fixed posture		50%
Kneeling or crouching		
Sitting		
Leg room sufficient		
Leg room insufficient or very limited		
Leg room non-existent		
Note:	Described time of lower limbs posture	100%

FIGURE 10.23 Quick assessment of postures of the lower limbs.

Use of lower limbs		
No pedals used		100%
Lower limbs used to press pedals		
Note:	Duration of lower limb use	100%

FIGURE 10.24 Quick assessment of postures: use of the lower limbs.

BIOMECHANICAL OVERLOAD FROM AWKWARD POSTURES - TRUNK AND LOWER LIMBS	
SUMMARY OF PRE-ASSESSMENT AND INTERVENTION PRIORITIES	Risk assessment necessary
	Risk assessment advisable as soon as possible.

FIGURE 10.25 Final summary of the quick assessment of postures of the trunk and lower limbs.

In this example, the postures are always standing but the lower limbs are stationary 50% of the time (while splitting off the slabs), and the worker can walk around inside (or even outside) the workshop the rest of the time.

It is worth noting that the lower limbs never operate pedals (Figure 10.24) and that at the bottom of the page, there is a summary of the pre-assessment of postures of the trunk and lower limbs with an indication of priorities (Figure 10.25).

10.2.5 PART 5: POLLUTANTS

As the *key enter* for pollutants was checked, the corresponding *quick assessment* work sheet for the presence of dust and particles needs to be completed.

Unlike for many chemicals, for which a technical data sheet and hazard labeling is usually available, there is no such reference to the potential toxicity of dust produced during slab cutting in this case. However, it is known that serpentine stone contains free silica and occasional traces of asbestos fibers. In the work sheet assessing the danger and toxicity of pollutants in the workplace, the indication is of "high toxicity" due to the presence of dust (Figure 10.26).

As regards the type and frequency of exposure (Figure 10.27), since there is no way to control the presence of dust, the work sheet indicates that the dust disperses "openly" in the workplace and that the quantities present are generally "high and daily".

Lastly, at the bottom of the page, there is a summary of the pre-assessment of chemical–physical pollutants in the workplace, as well as an indication of intervention priorities (Figure 10.28). In this example, a qualitative–quantitative instrumental analysis should be carried out to check for the presence of silica and potentially asbestos fibers.

10.2.6 PARTS 6 AND 7: BIOLOGICAL AGENTS AND STRESS

As already stated, these sections were not completed as no such problems were reported.

DUST / Silica				
	H300 H310 H330	VERY TOXIC		EXTREMELY HIGH
	H301 H311 H331	TOXIC		HIGH
	H314 H318	CORROSIVE		
	H302 H312 H332	HARMFUL		MEDIUM
	H315 H319 H335	IRRITATING		LOW
	H317 H334	SENSITIZING		SENSITIZATION RISK
X	H340 H350 H360	CARCINOGENIC; MUTAGENIC; REPRODUCTIVE CYCLE RISK; TERATOGENIC		EXTREMELY HIGH
	H341 H351 H361 H370 H372	CARCINOGENIC; MUTAGENIC; REPRODUCTIVE RISK; TERATOGENIC; TOXIC		HIGH
	H371 H373	TOXIC		MEDIUM
	H315 H319 H335 OR WITHOUT "H" LABEL	IRRITATING		LOW
	H317 H334	SENSITIZING		SENZITIZATION RISK
	H200 H201 H202 H203 H240 H241	EXPLOSION		
	H220 H222 H224 H241 H242 H251 H252	EXTREMELY FLAMMABLE		EXTREMELY HIGH
	H250	COMBUSTIBLE		
	H225 H228	EASILY FLAMMABLE		HIGH
	H204	EXPLOSIVE		
	H223 H226 (IN CERTAIN CONDITIONS) H225: se punto di	FLAMMABLE		MEDIUM
	NO LABEL	HIGH FLASH POINT (I.E. >70")		LOW

Health risks from acute exposure; Health risks from chronic exposure; Safety risks

FIGURE 10.26   Quick assessment of chemical and physical pollutants: toxicity and hazard.

	BRIEF DESCRIPTION OF THE MANUFACTURING PROCESS IN ORDER TO CHARACTERIZE WORKER EXPOSURE					
	TYPE OF EXPOSURE			FREQUENCY OF EXPOSURE		
	CLOSED CYCLE	CONTROLLED CYCLE	OPEN CYCLE	OCCASIONAL (not every day)	LOW BUT DAILY	HIGH AND DAILY
	COMPLETE	INHALATION/SEPARATIO N??	DIRECT CONTACT AND HANDLING			
DUSTS Silica			X			X

FIGURE 10.27 Quick assessment of chemical and physical pollutants: type of use and frequency of exposure.

SUMMARY OF PRE-ASSESSMENT AND INTERVENTION PRIORITIES	Risk assessment necessary
	to be evaluated as soon as possible

FIGURE 10.28 Final summary of quick assessments of pollutants.

10.2.7 Part 8: Summary of Results

This work sheet summarizes and graphically depicts the results obtained in the various sections of the pre-assessment of risk factors for the homogeneous group examined.

The results are entered automatically into the software as the various sections are completed.

The first part of the work sheet shows the biomechanical overload conditions (Figure 10.29, first section). The colors (present only in the software but not shown here) and the percentages generated indicate intervention priorities for each aspect of the biomechanical overload.

Another similar section follows, presenting the results of the analysis of all the other risk factors (Figure 10.29, second section), mainly through *key questions*, and with an actual *quick assessment* only for chemical–physical pollutants, biological agents and stress.

In conclusion, a summary is provided in the form of histograms whose height (from 0% to 100%) expresses the results in terms of priorities, thus creating a "risk profile" for the homogeneous group (Figure 10.30).

B	CHECK / IDENTIFICATION OF PRIORITIES FOR BIOMECHANICAL OVERLOAD		
B1	BIOMECHANICAL OVERLOAD OF UPPER LIMBS IN REPETITIVE TASKS	Present	100%
B2	BIOMECHANICAL OVERLOAD - MANUAL LOAD LIFTING AND ADDITIONAL ENVIROMENTAL RISK FACTORS	Present	100%
B3	BIOMECHANICAL OVERLOAD - MANUAL LOAD CARRYING	Present	100%
B4	BIOMECHANICAL OVERLOAD - MANUAL PULLING AND PUSHING AND ADDITIONAL ENVIROMENTAL RISK FACTORS	Present	65%
B5	BIOMECHANICAL OVERLOAD - AWKWARD POSTURES OF SPINE AND LOWER LIMBS	Present	60%
	CHECK / IDENTIFICATION OF PRIORITIES FOR OTHER WORKING CONDITIONS		
C	INDOOR LIGHTING PROBLEMS		0%
D	OUTDOOR WORK-RELATED PROBLEMS - UV RADIATION		25%
E	NOISE		75%
F	MICROCLIMATE PROBLEMS		50%
G	PROBLEMS ARISING FROM EQUIPMENT USE		100%
H	PROBLEMS RELATED TO VIBRATIONS		0%
I	MACHINERY-RELATED PROBLEMS		
J	ISSUES RELATED TO POLLUTANTS		100%
K	ISSUES RELATED TO BIOLOGICAL POLLUTANTS		0%
L	STRESS - ORGANIZATION		0%

FIGURE 10.29   Final summary work sheet: aspects concerning biomechanical overload and "other" risks.

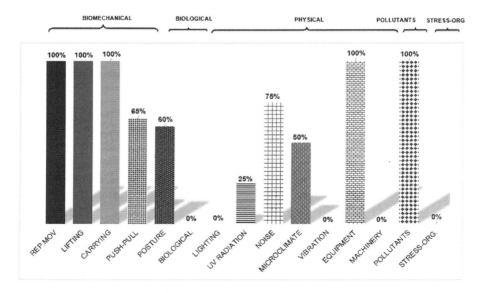

FIGURE 10.30   Final summary work sheet: results depicted in graphic form.

It is also worth noting that a specific data strip in the software highlights the results to be transferred to another software program for mapping multiple homogeneous groups in a given company or manufacturing sector, as shown in Figure 10.31.

REP.MOV	LIFTING	CARRYING	PUSH-PULL	POSTURE	BIOLOGICAL	LIGHTING	UV RADIATION	NOISE	MICROCLIMATE	VIBRATION	EQUIPMENT	MACHINERY	POLLUTANTS	STRESS-ORG.
100%	100%	100%	65%	60%	0%	0%	25%	75%	50%	0%	100%	0%	100%	0%

FIGURE 10.31 Final summary work sheet: indication of results to be transferred to other mapping work sheets.

11 Using ERGOCHECK for Pre-mapping Risk
Application Examples

CONTENTS

This chapter presents the results of the pre-mapping assessment performed in certain specific manufacturing sectors and representing some of the most common tasks that can be found in small and craft businesses, with excerpts from an article published in the Italian occupational medicine journal *Medicina del Lavoro* (Colombini et al., 2011), updated where necessary. Given their distinctive nature, it seemed appropriate to include these detailed organizational studies again here, first of all in order to better understand the work cycle, this being an essential step towards conducting an actual assessment of workplace discomfort and danger, albeit at the preliminary level. Even the mere identification of homogeneous groups to be analyzed requires an accurate understanding of the tasks and how they are distributed assignment within the homogeneous group(s).

11.1 LEATHERWORKING FOR THE PRODUCTION OF HANDBAGS

Giuseppina Coppola and Loretta Montomoli (†)
Reumatologia dell'Università di Siena

11.1.1 INTRODUCTION

In Italy, the leatherworking sector plays a fundamental role among small- and medium-sized enterprises; it belongs to what is known as the "Italian fashion system", underpinning which, in addition to leather goods, is the tanning industry, as well as textiles and apparel. Over recent years, the leatherworking sector has witnessed a gradual decline in volumes due to the transfer of upstream production processes to other parts of the world. As a result, the sector is now thriving in developing countries such as China, to the detriment of small- and medium-sized Italian companies. Nevertheless, in recent years Italy has experienced a slow upswing in this sector. In particular, the glimmerings of a recovery began to appear in 2017, although problems still remain unresolved in many small- and medium-sized enterprises (due to lack of entrepreneurial skills, poorly organized manufacturing systems, lack of specialization in specific sectors, etc.); in particular, export sales have climbed (with an increase in value between January and October 2017). According to preliminary estimates drawn up by the research unit of the main association representing Italian manufacturing companies, Confindustria, turnover in the footwear, tanning, leather goods, fur, eyewear, gold, jewelry and textile sectors are currently trending upward at +3.2%. Italy is characterized by its numerous industrial districts, i.e. clusters of small towns operating and co-operating in the same sector. Leather goods and tannery districts are mainly located in the central and northern regions of the country, particularly in Tuscany, around the cities of Arezzo, Florence and Pisa (especially Santa Croce sull'Arno), Marche (Tolentino, near Macerata) and Veneto (Arzignano, near Vicenza). The district near Solofra (in the southern Italian province of Avellino) is also well known for its approximately 60 tanneries.

11.1.2 LEATHER PROCESSING TECHNOLOGY (MONTOMOLI ET AL., 2011)

The tanning and leatherworking industry is very old, dating back to the classical era and flourishing in the Middle Ages, along with the growth of tanners' guilds. The technology has evolved apace with progress in chemistry; however, alongside modern factories, there are still innumerable artisanal tanneries that produce top quality leather. There are countless uses for hide and leather, suffice it to mention footwear, handbags, gloves and furs. The main processing phases are illustrated below (Candura, 1991).

The tanning process consists of a series of treatments designed to transform animal skins into leather by various chemical and physical methods. The resulting hides and skins are the finished products and have the following characteristics: the leather is soft and supple and can be used to produce clothes or footwear. Leather is generally obtained by "mineral" tanning. Tougher and more compact hides are used mainly for producing the soles of shoes. In general, they are produced by "vegetable" tanning. Both hide and leather are obtained from the skin of the animal, in particular the area of the dermis that is richest in collagen fibers lying perpendicularly to the surface, called the papillary layer, which in tanning jargon is called the "grain". Tanning is a highly complex process due to the large number of steps involved, each of which involves entails specific risks.

The process of tanning comprises the following distinct stages: pre-tanning of the skins, storage of the green hides and chemicals, beam house operations, tanning, post-tanning operations, intermediate manufacturing processes and finishing.

11.1.2.1   Pre-tanning Operations

  a. **Pre-treatment of the skins:** After slaughtering and before tanning, the animal skins must be stored for a variable period of time and; therefore, special precautions must be taken in order to prevent putrefaction. The skins are therefore disinfected and treated with preservatives. Disinfectants remove most pathogenic organisms, while preservatives are designed to prevent putrefaction after slaughtering and before tanning, thus enabling the skins to be transported even over long distances and stored for prolonged periods of time. The most widely used curing agent in Italy and Europe is salt (sodium chloride). Hides can be wet salted in a brine tank or dry stacked for heavy skins: fresh salted. In countries where table salt is taxed, industrial salt is used, i.e. denatured with various additives such as sodium carbonate, naphthalene, camphor, orthophenol, pentachlorophenate, sodium or potassium dichromate, or sodium fluoride in varying amounts.

  b. **Storage of raw hides and chemicals:** This is the phase in which the hides are stored with the chemicals that will be used to process them. Raw hides and skins can be stored outdoors or indoors; in some cases, they are stored in cool rooms.

  c. **Beam house operations:** Hide preparation treatments, in tanning jargon, are also called beam house operations and consist in soaking, unhairing-liming, fleshing, decalcination or deliming, degreasing, bating and pickling.

     Beam house operations include all the wet processes in which the hides are soaked in liming drums or vats, where they come into contact with a series of liquid chemical solutions that separate the hair from the hides, tan, dye and oil and prepare them for the following phases. Some of these steps are purely mechanical (fleshing, splitting and unhairing).

  c1) Soaking consists in washing the preserved skins to remove impurities, dissolve and remove sodium chloride and solubilize globular proteins. It is carried out in drums, with water and sometimes also surfactants, to rehydrate the fibers. Enzymes with a mild proteolytic and lipolytic action are also widely used for dry-preserved skins. Soaking is fundamental because all subsequent processes will depend on the exchange of solutes present in different concentrations in the solution outside and inside the skin.

c2) The purpose of unhairing and liming is to chemically remove the epidermal layer of the skin, saponify the fats in order to remove them, solubilize residual globular proteins and swell the skin thanks to the formation of spaces between the fibers and increase the thickness and tautness of the skin, all of which will help the tanning agent to penetrate more effectively. Skins of animals with fur still attached are called pelts, while shaved hides are called skins. These operations are also carried out in drums containing sodium sulfide (sometimes also sodium sulfydrate) and slaked lime (calcium hydroxide), and in some cases, other products such as aliphatic amines and various mercaptans.

c3) Fleshing consists in removing particles of subcutaneous tissue still attached to the dermis, i.e. the flesh. The operation is carried out mechanically by means of fleshing machines, consisting of two rotating cylinders: one coated with hard rubber on which the skin is placed and another with sharp helical blades, which quickly removing the flesh.

c4) The decalcination or deliming process removes the lime residue still present on the fibers after previous processes, lowering the pH. Decalcinating or deliming products are acids or acid reactive salts that form calcium-soluble compounds. Strong or weak acids, acid reactive salts or carbon dioxide may be used. Boric, oxalic, sulfuric and formic acids are widely used. This operation is also carried out in drums and may produce hydrogen sulfide.

c5) Scouring (or degreasing) consists in the partial removal of the natural fats contained in the skin, as excessive amounts could produce tanning defects and uneven dyeing. Degreasing is carried out by treating the hides in the drum with water and various surfactants (anionic, cationic, non-ionic). After degreasing, the skins are rinsed with lukewarm water (35°C–37°C). Degreasing can also be performed mechanically by pressure. Degreasing with solvents is generally carried out when the hides are dry, i.e. on already tanned or partially tanned and dried skins, making the process more complicated and more expensive. "Bating" (or maceration) fully opens up the fiber structure after the calcination or liming phase. Macerating products are preparations containing proteolytic enzymes of pancreatic origin such as pepsin and trypsin. With this process, the collagen structure is partially loosened, making the dermis more porous.

c6) The purpose of pickling is to stop the maceration process through acidification, thus significantly lowering the pH level, so as to further facilitate the subsequent penetration of the tanning agents. The compounds used are organic acids (sulfuric acid, formic acid, lactic acid, etc.) and salts (sodium chloride added before the acids, to avoid swelling). This highly acidic treatment is carried out to prepare the skins for chrome tanning; for vegetable tanning, the treatment is less aggressive, in fact the term used is "acidification" not pickling. The acidification process is carried out in drums at room temperature, with the skins stirred for 1–2 hours and then left to rest overnight. By acidifying the skins, residual sulfides from the liming process are released, with the subsequent formation of hydrogen sulfide (H_2S). Systems have therefore been put in place to extract this gas from the drums and send it to a scrubber, where it is abated into a basic solution.

11.1.2.2   The Tanning Process

Tanning prevents the skin from decomposing, makes it resistant to acid, alkali, water and heat and improves its mechanical characteristics. Tanning processes are classified according to the type of tanning agent used or collagen bond formed. Tanning agents are divided into two basic categories: inorganic (used for mineral tanning) such as chrome, aluminum, iron, zirconium and organic (used for vegetable tanning) comprised mainly of tannins (synthetic or vegetable), as well as oils and aldehydes.

a. **Mineral tanning:** This process uses compounds of chromium, aluminum, zirconium and iron.

   a1) *Chrome tanning:* Chromium is by far the most widely used tanning agent for various reasons: the process is quick, simple and easy to control and it produces leather that offers particularly good thermal stability; it can also produce extremely versatile leathers, with superior characteristics compared to those made with other tanning agents, either mineral or vegetable. For this treatment, basic chrome sulfate with 33% basicity is used.

   At present, there are two types of chrome tanning: single bath and double bath.

   The single bath method is the most common and is always preceded by pickling. To ensure that the chrome has penetrated the skin completely a small cut is made and the whole cross section must be green. The next step is basification, which has the two-fold purpose of reducing the sulfuric acid that may be released when chromium salts are added and of producing a slow and gradual increase in the pH level, through the addition of basic (alkali) salt (sodium bicarbonate).

   The double bath chrome tanning process involves the use of a chroming bath and a reduction bath. The chroming bath contains dichromate, sulfuric acid or hydrochloric acid and sodium chloride. The skins remain in the bath until they acquire a yellow-orange color when cut at the thickest point. Sodium hydrosulfite, sodium thiosulfate, sulfite, bisulfite or other reducing agents and sulfuric acid are added to the subsequent reducing bath. The skin remains here until it becomes green when cut. The double bath tanning process is used only for certain types of skins (kid).

a2) *Aluminum tanning:* It is rarely used and only for particular types of glove leather and furs. If used alone, it produces white leather and skins. The most common compound is aluminum sulfate.

a3) *Zirconium tanning:* This process produces very white, very strong and resistant leather. Rarely used alone, it is more often employed as a re-tanning agent, after chrome tanning, to modify certain characteristics. Zirconium salts have a greater tanning effect than aluminum salts; zirconium sulfate and zirconium chloride are used in their natural state or partially converted to basic.

b. **Organic tanning:** Vegetable tanning is the oldest known form of tanning and has been used since prehistoric times; occurring in many plants, tannins (glycosidic products containing phenolic groups) are derived from the processing of trees and plants such as chestnut, mimosa and oak. The operations that precede organic tanning are very similar to those for mineral tanning.

b1) *Tannin tanning:* In ancient times, this process consisted in burying the skins with fragments of the bark of oaks or other conifers soaked in water, and digging them up after several months when the tanning was completed. Three tanning procedures are currently used: slow, fast and ultra-fast. *Slow tanning* involves stacking and treating the skins with tannins and leaving them in a pit for about 3 months. The *fast tanning* process involves first placing the skins in a vat and then in drums for about 2 weeks. The *ultra-fast tanning* process involves placing the skins only in drums for 48 hours. Tannin tanning is used mainly to produce leather for footwear. By using synthetic tannins and combinations of different vegetable plant, it is possible to obtain leather in different colors with different characteristics.

b2) *Oil, fat or suede tanning:* This tanning process produces suede leather. It uses fish oils, whose composition (unsaturated fatty acids) gives rise to oxyacids that react with the functional groups of collagen.

b3) *Formaldehyde and glutaraldehyde tanning:* Formaldehyde, sometimes used to obtain soft, white leather, is mainly used as a re-tanning agent in chrome tanning and as a pre-tanning agent in oil tanning. Today, due to its known carcinogenic properties, formaldehyde tends to be replaced by glutaraldehyde.

11.1.2.3 Post-tanning Operations

a. **Splitting:** A mechanical processing whereby thicker skins are split into a more valuable upper epidermal layer ("grain") and a lower dermal part ("crust"), which is used for various purposes. For fine leathers, this operation can be carried out prior to tanning because tanning a thinner skin enhances the grain. If this operation is performed after tanning, more crust will be produced. Crust can in turn be re-tanned to make less valuable leathers.

b. **Shaving:** This is another mechanical process that determines the thickness of leather, depending on subsequent processing steps.

c. **Re-tanning:** Skins are placed in drums to enhance the quality of the leather using various types of tanning agents. Chemicals such as formaldehyde, glutaraldehyde and synthetic tannins are used.

d. **Fat liquoring:** Natural and synthetic oils are used to achieve softer, more supple leather. The purpose of this process is to lubricate the internal fibers; without this process, after drying, the skins would be firm and the end product hard, stiff and with a tendency to break.

11.1.2.4   Intermediate Manufacturing Processes

In these processes, the skins are subjected to mechanical processing to dry, stretch and soften them before the chemical finishing phase. The processes are partly wet and partly dry. Wet processes include (a) sammying, (b) vacuum drying, (c) overhead chain drying, (d) rapier oven drying and (e) vertical frame drying. Dry processes include (a) staking, (b) dry milling and (c) dry buffing.

Sammying is a process in which the skins are mechanically squeezed and then partially dried with compressed air.

Drying reduces the water content of hides by around 10%–15% through various systems.

Staking softens the whole skin, while milling is a process whereby the skins are placed in dry steel drums to soften the leather and produce a particular grain.

Milling is used for nubuck or suede leathers and to correct any defects on the grain side.

Leather dyeing is carried out by placing the skins in drums and adding synthetic organic dyes, generally acid. Some colors require preliminary bleaching with oxidizing substances. In large tanneries, tanning and dyeing operations can be carried out simultaneously in the same drum (tanning dyeing). Often, "drum tests" are carried out before dyeing, fat liquoring and re-tanning, i.e. small pieces of leather and other products are placed inside special "drums" to check and, if necessary, correct the amount of chemicals to be introduced into the drum together with the entire batch. Before drum tests, the skins are tested in a laboratory where chemical and physical testing is performed on samples.

11.1.2.5   Finishing

Finishing is comprised of several operations in order to create the best possible leather from a commercial standpoint. Therefore, it is the process featuring the greatest technological developments in tanning. A series of chemical and physical processes take place in the finishing phase to ensure that tanned leathers present the superior qualities called for by an increasingly demanding market, and where ever-changing cutting-edge methods are developed. Tanned hides are in fact coated with an impressive variety and number of chemical substances that are deposited on the surface in the form of films. Thus applied, the mixtures impart particular characteristics such as gloss, softness, elasticity, water resistance and wear resistance.

Finishing operations include *pigment coating, curtain coating, roller coating* and *padding.*

  a. *Pigment coating* is a surface treatment that colors and/or coats the skins. The pigment is applied by spray gun and the material is then sent to a drying tunnel.
  b. *Curtain coating* distributes a thin layer of dye. Thus coated, the skins are then placed to dry on racks in a heated room. The curtain coating machine is commonly used because one application produces the equivalent of 4–5 spray applications of coating mixtures. This technique is used primarily for painted leather, for which reactive paints are used, i.e. paints that leave a film by chemical reaction. There are two components, and the mechanism of action is based on the poly-addition of di-isocyanates. One of the two components is an isocyanate and the other is an organic polyester or polyether, i.e. a compound containing two or more hydroxyl alcohol groups per molecule.
  c. In *roller coating*, the surface of the leather is colored by contact with a cylinder over which the treatment product is distributed.
  d. *Padding* can be performed manually or mechanically. Manual padding is carried out only in some specialized tanneries and is designed to create nuances and/or shading on the leather; the pad is soaked in the coating mixture and passed over the skin. The padding machine, on the other hand, consists of a conveyor belt, spray gun, pads and a drying tunnel. Leather finishing also involves the use of various chemical substances, some of which (such as polyurethane in varnishes) give the product particular physical characteristics. There are various types of finishing, besides polyurethane: casein, in particular for shoe leather; aniline, in particular for fine, naturally flawless leather; resin, used for leather with imperfections; nitrocellulose, typical of highly resistant leather, such as for waterproof boots, suitcases, saddlery effects and linings.
      Finishing is followed by final operations such as cropping and trimming.
  e. *Cropping* removes excess skin from the corners. It is carried out manually with scissors or a special tool called a billhook.
  f. *Trimming* evens out the ragged edges of the skin and is carried out using an electric edge trimmer.

11.1.2.6   Production of Ladies' Handbags
The process for manufacturing ladies' handbags can be broken down into three main steps: (a) mechanical processes for producing the materials, (b) assembly and (c) finishing.

  a. **Mechanical processes for producing the materials:** In this first stage of the process, the main processes include:
      a1) *Degreasing:* In some cases, the hides arrive directly from the tannery to the factory that produces the bags, so it is necessary to eliminate some of the tannery oils with surfactants.

a2) *Cutting of the pieces:* Generally speaking, a handbag is comprised of several leather parts of different shapes and sizes (in some cases up to 100). The leather is cut by means of a die-cutter.

a3) *Splitting:* This operation is designed to thin the skin by removing excess hide. The thickness of each individual piece is decided based on what it will be used for.

a4) *Skiving:* This process removes impurities from the surface of the various leather pieces and is carried out on a fleshing machine.

b. **Assembly:** The parts are assembled in three different steps:

b1) *Bonding:* This process is carried out using spray guns that apply water-based adhesive (with low solvent content) to the components (leather and internal fabrics).

b2) *Stiffening:* Production of reinforced parts of the bag by stiffening, i.e. gluing more material to the parts bonded together in the previous step.

b3) *Sewing:* This step is carried out by means of sewing machines, some of which have attachments for zippers. The parts are first sewn then internally *glued.*

c. **Finishing processes:** The final step in the production of women's handbags may involve to color the edges, to attach handles and zips (previously glued) and trims. All these phases are carried out by hand or with a sewing machine.

11.1.3 COMPANIES INCLUDED IN THE ANALYSIS AND DEFINITION OF HOMOGENEOUS GROUPS

A total of three leatherworking companies were analyzed: a tannery, an intermediate manufacturing processing company and a manufacturer of ladies' handbags (referred to as "leather factory A and B").

Leather factory "A" prepares semi-finished products. The materials it works with (leather, imitation leather, fabric, etc.) are supplied directly by the fashion house. The manufacturing cycle includes the various phases described above, to provide the styles and types of products ordered, so the product being made reflects the latest trends in the fashion industry and the changing seasonal collections.

Leather factory "B" receives materials that are generally already cut, and the company assembles the parts and creates the finished bag. Here too, the type of work, the fabrics, the finishes and the work schedules all depend on the articles ordered by the fashion house.

The evaluation was carried out using the pre-mapping work sheet for identifying discomfort and dangers present in small and craft businesses. In each company, an inspection was carried out together with the occupational health physician and the production manager: every manufacturing process was filmed.

It was possible to break down the working population into homogeneous groups based on gender and task (Table 11.1). Since the employees were assigned to several tasks at the same time according to production requirements, it was possible to identify and form one homogeneous group per company.

TABLE 11.1

Breakdown of Employees by Task and Gender in the Three Companies Analyzed and Definition of the Three Homogeneous Groups

Breakdown of Tannery Work	No. Female Workers	No. Male workers
Buffing, milling and trimming	4	2
Leather ironing and sorting	4	
Finishing	6	15
Pressing, splitting and shaving		8
Wet blue department		1
Tanning		4
Sammying, vacuum drying and staking		8
Dyeing		4
Skiving		3
Tannery testing		1
Breakdown of Work at Leather Factory "A"	**No. Female Workers**	**No. Male Workers**
Warehouse and materials handling	12	3
Splitting and skiving	1	1
Gluing	3	
Bench work (finishing)	5	1
Sewing	3	1
Packaging	1	
Breakdown of Work at Leather Factory "B"	**No. Female Workers**	**No. Male Workers**
Sewing	4	
Assembly		1
Bench work (gluing, finishing)	4	1
Dyeing		1
Polishing		1
Leather goods/other	2	
Packaging	1	

11.1.4 RESULTS OF PRELIMINARY STUDIES: HAZARD ANALYSIS AND BIOMECHANICAL RISK "QUICK ASSESSMENT" MODELS FOR SETTING EVALUATION PRIORITIES USING THE ERGOCHECK WORK SHEET

11.1.4.1 The Tannery

In the tannery, the ERGOCHECK analysis revealed the presence of evaluation priorities for biomechanical factors (repetitive movements, lifting and awkward postures), organizational factors and physical factors such as microclimate, noise, tools and machinery (Figure 11.1). With regard to chemicals, large quantities of which are always present, the analysis generated a recommendation to carry out an

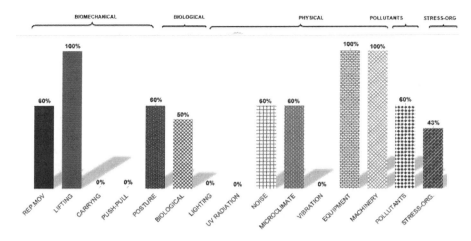

FIGURE 11.1 Summary of the results of the pre-mapping assessment of the homogeneous group of tannery workers.

evaluation, which was, however, not urgent. This may be due to a lack of sufficient information regarding all the chemicals used (safety data sheets), thus preventing the pre-mapping work sheet from being correctly applied.

11.1.4.2   Intermediate Manufacturing Processes

With regard to the companies carrying out the intermediate operations (indicated, respectively, as A and B), the histograms depicting the results of the pre-mapping assessment reveal several intervention priorities and, above all, conditions featuring different levels of severity.

Company A, represented by the histogram in Figure 11.2a, is especially in need of an evaluation for repetitive movements of the upper limbs, biomechanical overload due to manual load lifting, and pushing and pulling. In this case, there is no doubt that the evaluation of pollutants is necessary and must be monitored, as it derives from an analysis of all the technical data sheets present in the company.

Figure 11.2b shows the results of the intermediate manufacturing processes present in Company B; its characteristics are more similar to those of the tannery and evaluation priorities were detected for biomechanical factors (critical for repetitive movements and lifting), organizational factors and physical factors such as microclimate, noise, tools and machinery. Here too, the analysis of pollutants, which highlighted the need for evaluation with intervention recommended but not urgent, was undermined by the lack of reliable data concerning the substances used.

11.1.4.3   Production of Ladies' Handbags

Both companies making women's handbags generated histograms (Figure 11.3a and b) showing a clear prevalence of the risk of biomechanical overload of the upper limbs (i.e. evaluation necessary as soon as possible) and of the risk deriving from

(a) Summary of pre-mapping assessment for Company A: homogeneous group performing intermediate manufacturing processes

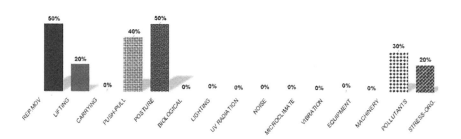

(b) Summary of pre-mapping assessment for Company B: homogeneous group performing intermediate manufacturing processes

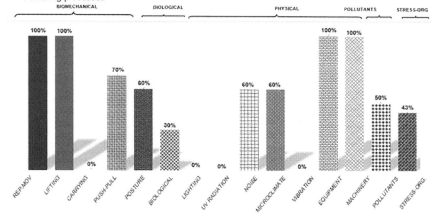

FIGURE 11.2 (a) and (b) Summary of the results of the pre-mapping assessment of intermediate manufacturing processes in Companies A and B.

tools (injuries due to sharp objects). Moreover, it should be noted that in Company A, there is a need to evaluate the pulling and pushing tasks. This company, unlike the Company B, has a much more complex manufacturing cycle that also involves transporting very large hides on trolleys, to be cut before moving on to subsequent phases.

With regard to the risk of exposure to environmental pollutants, the assessment indicates that intervention is recommended but not high priority because the list of chemicals in use (particularly non-aromatic polycyclic hydrocarbons) was comprehensive but not exhaustive, as there was no information on toxicity, harmfulness and flammability, with a likely underestimation of their extent.

(a) Summary of pre-mapping assessment in company A: homogeneous group involved in the production of women's bags

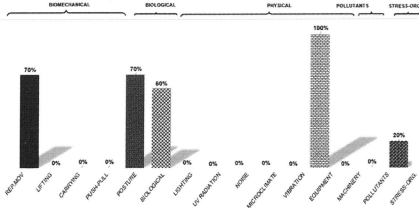

(b) Summary of pre-mapping assessment in company A: homogeneous group involved in the production of women's bags

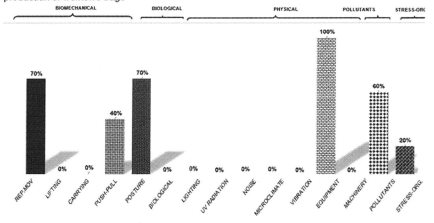

FIGURE 11.3 (a) and (b) Summary of the results of the pre-mapping assessment for womens' handbag manufacturing processes in Companies A and B.

11.1.5 Conclusions

The pre-mapping work sheet for identifying discomforts and danger in the workplace has produced a preliminary overview of all the main risk factors present in the leatherworking industry.

Despite carrying out the analysis on a limited group of companies, the work cycle involved in the production of artisanal (but high fashion) women's handbags has been analyzed as a whole.

The method appears to offer employers a useful tool for instantly highlighting priorities for intervention in respect of individual risk factors.

In this particular case, the pre-assessment work sheets showed that in the leather-working industry the risk of biomechanical overload of the upper limbs (repetitive movements) and the spine (lifting, pulling and pushing) is not only present, but reaches levels that in many cases calls for an urgent evaluation (or intervention).

Moreover, in the two homogeneous groups represented by the tannery and Company B (intermediate manufacturing), there are also obvious risks deriving from the organization of the work (rather than from stress) and from exposure to physical agents such as noise and microclimate.

With regard to the risk posed by chemical pollutants, all the companies assessed presented conditions in which remedial actions or interventions were recommended but not a priority. As already stated, this seems to be due to a lack of information on the chemicals used, because the list of substances in use appeared not to be exhaustive in terms of both qualitative and quantitative information, determining the likely underestimation of the risks.

11.2   USING THE PRE-MAPPING WORK SHEET TO ASSESS HAZARDS IN THE DECORATIVE CERAMICS SECTOR

Giorgio Di Leone
Area North ASL Bari

11.2.1   INTRODUCTION

Decorative ceramics are part of the larger ceramic production industry, which has been studied for some time now in relation to various occupational risks, ranging from noise to biomechanical overload, exposure to crystalline free silica and the alleged carcinogenic risk associated with ceramic fibers in the production of crockery, sanitary ware and so on.

Decorative ceramics occupy more of a "niche" sector, characterized by four types of manufacturers, as per data supplied by the Italian Federation of Italian craft enterprises (Confartigianato Imprese, 2008):

- Artistic commercial enterprises: Larger in size and able to readily cope with even very large orders.
- Artistic craft enterprises: With up to 15 employees. These are high-quality companies with a widespread distribution network.
- Traditional artistic businesses: Almost exclusively serving local markets. These small workshops produce very high-quality products and are innovation-driven.
- Semi-finished ceramic manufacturers: These companies produce high-quality garden pottery and semi-finished products for the hobby market.

The first Italian Conference on Artistic Ceramics, held in Rome in October 2008 (ARTEX, 2008), pointed out that there were about 3,000 companies operating in the sector in Italy in 2006 (located throughout the entire country, but mainly in the Emilia Romagna region), employing over 10,000 people (although the trend was decreasing). The situation has not changed radically since then. Italy is the leading country in the international ceramic trade, accounting for 40% of total volumes and turnover.

Unlike the rest of the ceramics industry, no free crystalline silica or ceramic fibers are reported in the decorative ceramics sector, and the most likely occupational risk is associated with biomechanical overload of the upper limbs and spine. Nonetheless, there could be exposure to chemicals used in the enamels and paints with which the products are decorated.

According to figures reported by INAIL (the Italian workers' compensation authority) (INAIL, 2009), and the regional authorities, in 2009, there were 695 reported cases of osteoarticular, muscular and connective tissue disorders in the decorative ceramics sector between 1992 and 2008 (Table 11.2 and Figure 11.4).

The most common disorders involved the tendons, joints and bursae, muscles, ligaments, fascia and soft tissues.

The amount of available data has been growing over the last few years, in line with the rising trend in the reporting of work-related disorders and diseases. The characteristics and dimensions of the sector, prevalently comprised of craft and small businesses, and the frequency with which pathologies involving the muscles, tendons, and ligaments are being reported, led to the decision to test the pre-mapping assessment software on the discomforts and dangers present among workers (Di Leone et al., 2011).

TABLE 11.2

Claims for Occupational Diseases of the Osteoarticular System Muscles and Connective Tissue in the Field of Artistic Ceramics in the Period 1992–2008

Musculoskeletal Occupational Diseases	Temporary	Permanent	Without Compensation	Negative	Total
Osteoarthritis and related diseases	2	11	1	40	54
Other lesions and joint manifestations	–	3	4	2	9
Disorders of intervertebral discs	–	20	3	46	69
Tendon diseases and diseases of the synovials, tendons and bursae	50	82	36	172	340
Disorders of muscles, ligaments, aponeuroses and soft tissues	37	49	34	80	200
Osteocondropaties	1	–	–	–	1
Flat foot and acquired deformations of the toes	–	–	–	1	1
Other osteomuscular disorders	1	4	2	14	21
Total	91	169	80	355	695

Source: INAIL (2009).

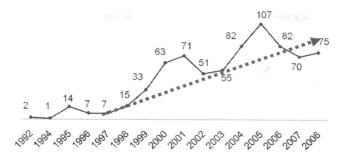

FIGURE 11.4   Claims for occupational diseases of the osteoarticular system, muscles and connective tissue in the field of artistic ceramics in the period 1992–2008. Distribution by year of the event. (INAIL, 2009.)

11.2.2   Organizational Analysis of the Sector

The raw material used to produce ceramics is clay, which is supplied (wet) in bags weighing 25 kg, delivered on a single pallet, unloaded by fork-lift truck and deposited at the entrance of the factory. Some or all of the workers then stack the bags in the workshop.

The work of producing ceramics is performed by the potter, fire master (or setter) and decorator (Figure 11.5). Sometimes there is also a general laborer, who mainly transports materials during the various phases of the manufacturing process and carries out minor finishing operations (for example, eliminating excess clay to ensure smooth edges of tiles, etc.).

11.2.2.1   The Work of the Potter

The production cycle begins with the degassing of the clay, to free it from any residual intrinsic gaseous components and thus enhance its technical characteristics. The clay is removed from the bag, "sliced" into several pieces around 2-cm thick and

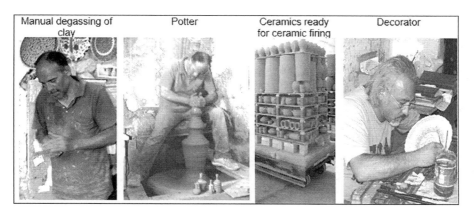

FIGURE 11.5   Some examples of main tasks performed in the preparation of artistic ceramics.

placed in a mixer to facilitate the elimination of residual gas. It then goes through a low-pressure chamber to remove even more gas and is finally extruded in the form of a cylindrical paste which, suitably cut, becomes the actual raw material. In craft companies with a strong focus on decorative ceramics, the potter works the pieces of clay (each one roughly the size of a coconut) manually, molding and slapping them until each piece acquires a compact and approximately spherical shape.

Throwing (working on the potter's wheel or lathe) is the most delicate phase, which gives the product the required shape. In more traditional settings, the wheel is operated by pedal, which controls the speed according to the thrust given to the lower flywheel. In many workshops, traditional wheels have been replaced by motorized ones controlled by a pedal clutch. In both cases, the most challenging part of the task is performed by the upper limbs, which are wholly engaged (from shoulder to fingers) to give the clay the desired shape. The greatest biomechanical overload involves the shoulders, especially in the initial phase, during which the potter applies the greatest pressure to the clay to begin shaping and thinning it. The pressure exerted by the hands gives the rotating mass of clay the characteristic shape that the object will ultimately have.

In this phase, the operator uses precise, delicate and highly skilled movements, combining strength (firm but not rough) with sensitivity, to give the clay the desired shape and thickness. Lastly, a suitably shaped spatula (crescent-shaped, and with a different radius depending on the design of the object) is used to smooth the surface and remove any wrinkles produced during the throwing operations. A steel wire is used to cut the object off at the base (a particularly skilled operator leaves only a very thin film of clay on the wheel), freeing it from the machine. At this point, the same operator moves the product (at this stage, defined as "green") from the wheel to a drying surface. Particularly large products sometimes require two workers: given the plasticity of wet clay, mishandling could damage the object and cause it to lose its shape.

If necessary, before firing, various decorations or details (also made out of clay) are added in order to create the final object: in some cases, these tasks can take the better part of the working day, considering the very wide range of products made (from a simple jug to a doll, not to mention extremely complex designs such as sculptures).

11.2.2.2 The Work of the Fire Master (or Setter)

After drying, the ware is sent to the kiln for firing: the fire master supervises this phase. Several layers of bricks, suitably spaced according to the size and shape of the objects to be fired, are stacked or set to form shelves that support and contain the objects to be fired.

Electric or gas-fired kiln oven reach average temperatures of 1,000°C–1,400°C. After firing (which, depending on the kiln, can take from 8 to 18 hours, followed by at least 72 hours for cooling), the fire master will empty the kiln (an operation that takes an average of 30 minutes), readying the objects (bisque ware) for the next stage of glazing that is carried out with water-based primers, and mixing the various colors, according to the expertise of the individual workshop. This operation may be carried out by the decorator or by the fire master. After mixing and blending the paint in special containers, or basins, (an operation that in traditional workshops is not carried out using mechanical stirrers but using the hands, so that the worker can feel the ideal consistency of the glaze), the operator picks up each piece using special tongs and manually dips it into a glazing bath, coating it in a very thin layer (the blanket). Once the object has been removed, due to the porosity of the terracotta the primer dries very quickly so it can be handled almost immediately. The skill of the operator, at this stage, lies in preventing the glaze from settling while still wet, and avoiding drips or smears that would spoil the appearance of the finished product. Each piece takes about a minute to glaze, and this work takes up a good part of the fire master's working day.

The fire master also supervises the second firing of the product after decoration, using methods very similar to the first setting in the kiln: in this case, even greater expertise is required to optimize the use of the kiln, into which as many of the decorated objects as possible are placed, without wasting space or any of them touching, because otherwise their surfaces would meld into a single piece, and the whole batch would be wasted.

The objects coming out of the glazing bath are then touched up to eliminate any defects due to operator error (casting effects) and to eliminate the impression left by the tongs (which leave unglazed spots). These flaws are corrected using a spatula and a brush and must be carried out when the product is still wet (and can be handled by the operator), because excessive drying prevents the finished product from displaying the typical vitreous surface free of wrinkles or flaws. These corrections can be carried out by the fire master or decorator.

11.2.2.3   The Work of the Decorator

The most highly skilled operator, or the one with the greatest artistic flair, completes the piece before the second firing. In a seated, and often ergonomically awkward, position the decorator uses a brush to decorate each individual piece: obviously the decorator needs confidence and precision, because mistakes are not possible.

Depending on its size, each piece takes an average of 30 minutes to complete, and the decorator sometimes spends an entire day in the same position painting a large batch of pieces with similar or different decorations.

Lastly, the decorated product is re-fired (by the fire master), giving the ceramic ware a glazed appearance.

11.2.2.4   Packaging

The last phase in the process consists of wrapping the individual pieces (in bubble wrap) and placing into boxes.

About 30% of craft businesses carry out the complete manufacturing cycle; in most cases the initial phase (handling the clay sacks, throwing on the potter's wheel, drying and preliminary firing) is skipped, as semi-finished products produced by specialized artisan companies set up for this purpose are used. In such cases, the remaining processes involve only decorating the pieces (sometimes using decals), second firing and warehousing.

11.2.3   Pre-mapping Assessment, Companies and Homogeneous Groups

The pre-mapping work sheets for assessing discomfort and dangers in the workplace, as presented in this volume, were used to inspect three companies that produce decorative ceramics.

Company A, located in the province of Taranto, is comprised of four operators (including the owner). This company focuses primarily on the creative aspect, with the operators free to manage their own working hours. The type of work performed in this company, which is more artistic than artisanal, defies the traditional description of "tasks", and its manufacturing cycle includes all the steps typical of the production of decorative ceramics: storage of the raw material, manual degassing of the clay, throwing on a traditional lathe (with the flywheel operated by pedal), first firing, glazing (with the enamels mixed with bare hands inside plastic basins), manual decoration, second firing and final manual touch-ups. There are two specialized workers in this company, the potter and the decorator, and two generic workers, the fire master and the laborer. Even the working environment is extremely traditional, with 50% of the workspace situated inside a cave. Lighting and microclimatic conditions are problematic.

Company B, located in the southern Italian province of Lecce, and is comprised of eight workers (including the three owners). Here, besides the traditional processes described above, there is also a certain amount of automation: automatic degassing of the clay, motorized lathe, some types of products are made using an automatic press, automatic glaze mixing, mechanical touch-ups of the intermediate product. About 40% of the company's production is comprised of semi-finished articles that it sells to other companies that focus less on the creative aspect and that simply finish decorating them (often using decals). Therefore, the manufacturing cycle can be defined as "semi-industrial" and the way the work is organized places the accent on productivity, with many more stereotypic and repetitive task. The finished products are often quite large and may require the manual handling of heavy objects.

The work environment is modern, and the lighting and ventilation are better than in the previous factory, but there is more automation, causing noticeable effects and a higher risk of workplace accidents and harmful vibrations.

Company C, situated near Siena, is comprised of two partners, who carry out the various tasks involved in creating the finished product. The decoration is carried out by an outside artist and the manufacturing cycle is partly automated. The factory makes decorative terracotta products, as well as crockery, statues and vases of various sizes. The clay arrives in pre-formed blocks and the operators only have to shape it. The manufacturing cycle entails: cutting the block of clay to size (and placing any leftover bits into an automatic mixer), working some of the clay using industrial methods (an automatic press, revolving press and mechanical lathe), but also using artisanal methods (semi-automatic potter's lathe without a pedal) and creating objects from plaster casts. More specifically, this latter process is a very ancient one that involves pressing the clay manually into plaster casts of varying sizes and shapes depending on the object to be made. The clay remains in the case for about 24 hours. Before baking in the furnace, the object is dried at room temperature for about a week in summer and a month in winter. After that all the objects, regardless of what technique is used to make them, are fired in gas ovens at a temperature of approx. 700°C. Some objects, such as crockery, are glazed by being submerged in enamel baths. The objects are then re-fired.

In Companies A and B, the risk pre-mapping work sheet was filled in during joint inspections by a local health unit inspector, an occupational health physician and an industrial hygienist, and the information was provided by homogeneous groups of potters and decorators. Company C was inspected by an occupational health physician and education and training specialist. It was not possible to form homogeneous groups in Company C as all the workers performed all the tasks: the results therefore refer to the entire manufacturing process.

11.2.4 RESULTS OF THE PRE-MAPPING ASSESSMENT

11.2.4.1 The Potter: A Comparison Between the Pre-mapping Assessments of the Artistic-Artisanal Company (A) and the Semi-Industrial Company (B)

The work sheet for pre-mapping risks and discomfort for potters in Companies A and B produced the results that can be seen in the graphs depicted in Figure 11.6 (Company A and Company B).

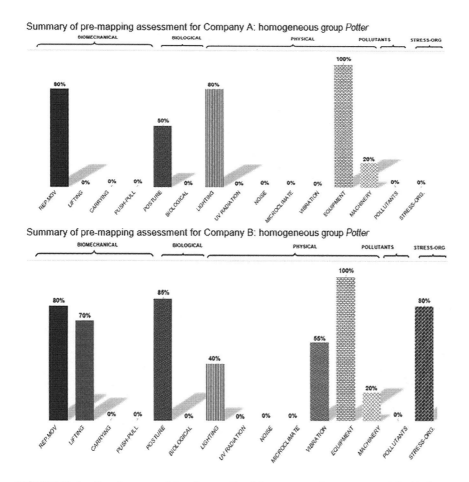

FIGURE 11.6 Graph summarizing the results of the pre-mapping assessment for the homogeneous group of potters in Company A and Company B.

There are significant differences between the results for the more "artistic" Company (A), calling for the "hazards" associated with repetitive movements and prolonged awkward postures to be explored in further depth, along with issues associated with poor lighting, and those of Company B, where there are also problems relating to manual load lifting, work pace and vibrations, but where the lighting is not as poor. Both companies also reported issues relating to the tools used for manually shaping the clay, with the risk of developing calluses, scratches, etc.

11.2.4.2 The Decorator: A Comparison Between the Pre-mapping Assessments of the Artistic-Artisanal Company (A) and the Semi-Industrial Company (B)

The results for the decorator are summarized in Figures 11.7 (Company A and Company B).

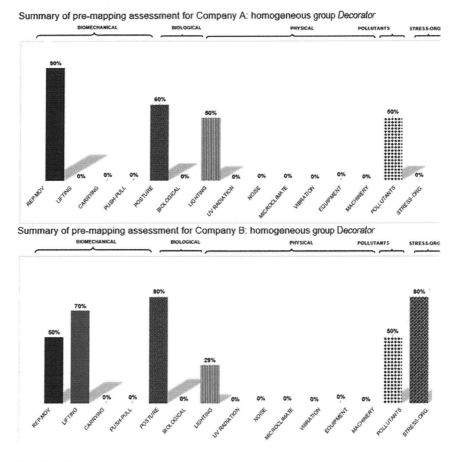

FIGURE 11.7   Graph summarizing the results of the pre-mapping assessment for the homogeneous group of decorators in Company A and Company B.

Here too there are significant differences. The decorators in Company A perform repetitive movements with their upper limbs and there is poor lighting; prolonged awkward postures are also mentioned. Pollutants in the form of dyestuffs and enamels/glazes are also present.

In Company B alongside these factors, there is also the manual handling of large finished products and sometimes a quite demanding work pace. Lighting is less of a problem. The second-level analysis quickly ruled out any risk associated with the use of chemicals. Indeed, through a more in-depth inspection of the toxicology work sheets, it was found that the factory used water-based dyestuffs, paints and enamels that were non-toxic, and in compliance with regulations and standards for crockery to be used for serving food.

11.2.4.3 Company C: Results of the Pre-mapping Assessment for Exposure of all Workers to all Tasks (One Only Homogeneous Group)

The graph summarizing the results for all tasks performed in Company C is indicated in Figure 11.8.

As mentioned above, the analysis of Company C refers to the entire manufacturing process, as the work is not organized on the basis of specialized skills and all the workers perform all the tasks. Repetitive movements of the upper limbs and awkward postures again emerge as priority issues, but the use of machinery and dust inhalation are also reported as potential risks.

11.2.5 DISCUSSION AND CONCLUSIONS

ERGOCHECK was found to be a useful tool for carrying out preliminary inspections and subsequently for investigating the discomfort and hazards present in all the workplaces. It is easy to use and helpful not only for employers and/or their health

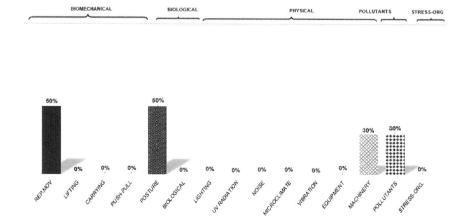

FIGURE 11.8 Graph summarizing the results of the pre-mapping assessment for the homogeneous group in Company C.

and safety consultants (who can use the work sheets to identify hazards calling for the appointment of an occupational health and safety physician even the risk evaluation phase) but also for helping occupational health and safety physicians to conduct inspections for the purposes of designing health surveillance protocols. Worker safety representatives can also use the program to identify and monitor hazardous workplace situations, as well as labor inspectors responsible for analyzing workplaces and assessing occupational risks.

As also shown by the variability in the results for the individual homogeneous groups examined in the different factories analyzed here, the work sheet has been proven to be very sensitive, insofar as it tends to overestimate hazards. However, this aspect should be viewed as an advantage, since it is desirable in the pre-mapping phase, for there to be greater sensitivity and lower specificity, in order to identify the aspects upon which to focus attention (so as to potentially remove them during the analytical risk assessment).

The decorative ceramics sector features certain peculiarities that give rise to the following considerations:

- Of all the various tasks, it is those of the potter and the decorator that warrant the greatest attention.
- The more "artistic" the production process, the greater the likelihood of workers being able to set their own pace and reduce stereotypies.
- Occupational risks are dramatically lower in companies that merely decorate the semi-finished products manufactured elsewhere. This work often involves the application of decals, so that even the decorator's work involves much less risk.
- In companies that produce semi-finished products and have less focus on the "artistic" aspects, the work pace may be faster and the workload heavier. In such environments, the indicators of potential risk for potters and decorators are more significant.

The pre-mapping assessment work sheet has thus proven to be sensitive enough to pick up the differences between manufacturing sites and pave the way for more in-depth investigations.

11.3   THE WORK OF THE DENTAL TECHNICIANS
Maurizia Giambartolomei

11.3.1   INTRODUCTION

In dental laboratories, the work of manufacturing and optimizing custom-made restorative and dental appliances, especially dentures, is carried out following the dentist's written and oral instructions.

All dental laboratories can carry out all the various tasks involved but, as a rule, there is a tendency for them to specialize due to the presence of a large number of small and very small laboratories with few employees and not always equipped with all the necessary equipment and machinery. Dental technicians therefore often concentrate on certain specific products depending on staff numbers, professional skills, available equipment and the needs of the dental practices with whom they work. For example, partial mobile dentures are generally manufactured in specialized laboratories that a certain number of small dental laboratories work with.

Larger laboratories usually carry out all their activities in-house. Some technicians may perform certain repetitive tasks for extended periods (e.g. milling, casting, etc.). In most small laboratories, technicians are not assigned to perform specific tasks, but rather, "everyone does everything" for short periods. Task diversification during the working day in small laboratories reduces the monotony of the job while sharing a common workplace exposes all operators to the same environmental risks.

Typically, the dentures or dental prosthetics are continuously passed from the dentist to the dental technician and vice versa, alternating clinical and laboratory work.

The dentist takes the impression containing information about the morphological details of the patient's oral cavity; this is a "negative impression" of the patient's mouth. The impression is sent to the dental laboratory which, depending on the type of prosthesis, starts the process of denture making, sometimes in collaboration with other laboratories. There may be multiple visits between the patient, dentist and dental laboratory.

The sector is characterized by the use of innovative and sometimes groundbreaking technologies and products, combined with a manufacturing system that is still largely artisanal and highly customized.

According to the most recent data, Italy has some 12,800 dental laboratories. The figures show that the number of dental laboratories is gradually decreasing, and that number of employees per company is generally low (1.68), one of the lowest in the EU and quite incomparable to the situation in the United Kingdom, where there are several hundred dental laboratories each with hundreds of employees. Based on information provided by CNA (*Confederazione Nazionale dell'Artigianato e della Piccola e Media Impresa* – the Italian Confederation of Crafts and Small and Medium Enterprises) in 2017, there were approximately 16,500 dental laboratories in Italy, of which 15,000 were very small businesses with a total of 27,000 employees.

The first "European Day of Dental Technicians" was held in June 2018, promoted by the FEPPD (*Fédération Européenne et Internationale des Patrons Prothésistes Dentaire*). The FEPPD represents 40,000 dental laboratories and 210,000 dental technicians across Europe. Italian data published on the ANTLO website (*Associazione Nazionale Titolari Laboratorio Odontotecnico* – National Association of Dental Laboratory Owners) indicate that there are 15,000 dental laboratories in Italy, employing about 23,000 people (ANTLO, 2018).

In terms of products, 89% of laboratories stated that they mainly make mobile partial dentures, 81% fixed prostheses in ceramic material, 57% fixed prostheses in resin.

Relatively "new" technologies have led to the disappearance of the partial removable denture in favor of mobile prostheses in thermoplastic material that require laboratories to be equipped with specific equipment such as special presses, crucibles and a 550°C muffle furnace.

Computerized technologies such as CAD/CAM (Computer-Aided Design/Computer-Aided Manufacturing) systems are particularly useful insofar as they are easy to use and produce accurate results, allowing for models to be scanned and data to be sent online to the machine tool.

In most EU countries, dental technicians are classified as an engineering profession. In Italy, it is classed as a technical profession. The latest classification of professions released by the Italian statistics bureau (ISTAT) reflects the innovations introduced by the International Standard Classification of Occupations and classifies dental technicians under "other technical health professions".

The mismatch between official data and actual data makes it difficult to determine the real dimensions of the sector in question: many more workers may in fact be exposed to occupational risks than those included in the current statistics. It is likely that the number of exposed workers is underestimated due to the presence of makeshift workplaces located in cramped spaces or rooms, even in dental practices, all too often devoid of personal protection equipment.

11.3.2   THE TECHNOLOGY CYCLE (GIAMBARTOLOMEI AND BOLOGNINI, 2011)

The next step is to describe the types of work and the different tasks that characterize them, along with the various materials, products and equipment used during the work phases (Figure 11.9).

11.3.2.1   The Main Tasks Common to the Different Types of Work

The dental laboratory is characterized by several different types of work, making for a very complex scenario. The restoration or reconstruction of missing or damaged teeth is one such job, along with the aesthetic and functional enhancement of the chewing process. Based on the design and specific indications received from the dentist, the dental technician painstakingly produces prosthetic appliances that may be mobile (removable) or fixed. The mobile appliances range from traditional complete dentures and metal partial dentures that replace individual teeth, to removable appliances held in place by implants. Fixed appliances include restorations on a single element or bridge, cemented to teeth reduced to a stump by the dentist, or to implants. There are also repairs of both fixed and mobile prostheses.

Certain activities are common to almost all technological cycles and are repeated to produce each individual product. These are the initial and final activities of the processes: sanitizing, casting, trimming, positioning on the articulator, sandblasting, degreasing, finishing and polishing.

11.3.2.2   Equipment

The equipment that can be found in a dental laboratory may vary and depends on the type of appliances produced and the size of the business.

In the dental laboratory, dental plaster, Bunsen burners, hand tools such as cups and spatulas, cutters and drills, waxes and muffle furnaces are the basic tools required

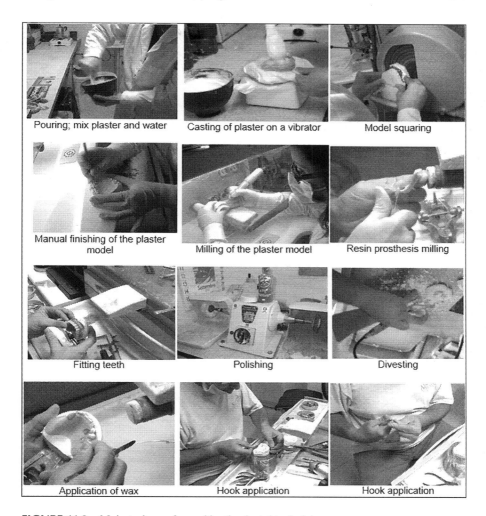

Pouring; mix plaster and water	Casting of plaster on a vibrator	Model squaring
Manual finishing of the plaster model	Milling of the plaster model	Resin prosthesis milling
Fitting teeth	Polishing	Divesting
Application of wax	Hook application	Hook application

FIGURE 11.9 Main tasks performed by the dental technician.

to carry out the main tasks involved. In addition, the following is a non-exhaustive list of equipment that can generally be found in a dental laboratory: pressure and UV polymerization machines, trimmers, fume extractor hoods, localized exhaust fans, articulators, duplicators, ovens and casting rings, polishers, vaporizers, dental wax melters, vibrators, presses, welding machines and pneumatic chisels.

11.3.2.3 Summary of Tasks by Finished Product

The main tasks performed in a dental laboratory, as described above, regardless of the finished product, are now listed again in Table 11.3 but on the basis of the finished product.

TABLE 11.3

Summary of Tasks Broken Down by Finished Product

Skeletal Prosthetic Production (Skeleton)

*The skeleton is a mobile partial prosthesis, made of chrome / cobalt / molybdenum, which exploiting
the elasticity of this alloy allows it to be hooked to natural teeth by means of cast hooks.*

Prosthesis Production (Fixed and/or Mobile)

*After sanitizing the impressions, casting with plaster and squaring the model, the wax model is then
made, which is poured with refractory material and placed in an oven at 400°C–900°C with
elimination of the wax (lost wax). Subsequently, the model is inserted into the casting machine and
the base of the product is made through the introduction of the metal alloy. Sandblasting and finishing
of the model and ceramic or resin coating operations follow. The ceramic alloy is applied to the metal
product and placed in the oven.*

*In the muffle process, the wax is spread, it is inserted into the muffle, and the model is duplicated. The
excess wax is then eliminated with boiling water and steam. In the polymerization process, the resin
is modeled and the polymerization is repeated several times, the dentine is finished, the enamel is
applied and the polymerizer is placed again. The final finishing and polishing follow.*

Orthodontic Prosthesis Production

Combined Prosthesis Production

Fixed Prosthesis Repair

Repair Mobile Prosthesis

11.3.3 DEFINITION OF HOMOGENEOUS GROUPS

The laboratory under examination mainly produces mobile dentures; attention
is devoted to providing the dentist with orthodontic and gnathological support.
Orthodontics is that branch of dentistry that studies abnormalities in the formation,
development and position of the teeth contained in the maxillary bones. Its purpose
is to prevent, eliminate or mitigate these abnormalities by maintaining or restor-
ing the teeth and facial profile in the most correct position possible. Gnathology is
the branch of dentistry that studies the physiology, pathologies and functions of the
masticatory system (including swallowing, voice and postural disorders); therefore, it
also studies the relationships between the upper and lower jaws, teeth, right and left
temporomandibular joints, the muscles that move the jaws and the nervous system
that controls those muscles, including the tongue.

The laboratory under examination does not perform tempering, melting or acid
pickling operations. They occasionally make partial dentures that are usually pur-
chased from other laboratories.

The quantities produced annually, broken down into cycles, are as follows: 30%
mobile prosthetic appliances, 15% orthodontic appliances, 15% repairs, 20% fixed
dentures, 10% partial dentures and 10% combinations. The laboratory has started to
set itself up to make appliances out of thermoplastic resins.

Three people work in the laboratory: the owner and two employees.

The work is organized as follows: the three operators work 5 days a week for
8 hours a day, during which there is always a 30-minute meal break, plus 2 coffee

breaks lasting 10 minutes each, one mid-morning and another mid-afternoon (the owner takes only one coffee break).

The owner also mans the phone and carries out visual inspections. The employees spend about 20 minutes a day cleaning the tools and equipment.

The owner carries out specific orthodontic tasks such as preparing fixed appliances, fabricating hooks and clasps; waxing, inserting and assembling teeth for the fabrication of complete removable and fixed dental prostheses. He also performs the final polishing of the products. Working in conjunction with the dentist takes up about 20% of the total working time of the dental technician who owns the company. He also devotes part of his time to being "on call" for any urgent modifications or corrections, and therefore is often called upon by his staff to perform finishing tasks in the dental lab.

The tasks of the two employees mainly involve disinfecting, casting models out of plaster and water, trimming and positioning the model on the articulator, milling and finishing operations, and divesting the mold from around a casting.

Having observed how the tasks are distributed, two homogeneous groups were identified: one comprised of the owner and other of the two employees.

11.3.4 Results of Preliminary Studies: Analysis of Discomfort and Hazards by Applying Pre-mapping Work Sheets

In order to analyze the dental technician's laboratory, a single pre-mapping work sheet has been compiled relating to the general discomfort and hazards involved due to the fact that both homogeneous groups share the same working environment, which is small (about 38 m^2), and that certain specific processes are not performed in enclosed spaces will walls up to the ceiling but by low room dividers.

Based on observations, the work cycles revealed no hazards connected with manual load handling, while there were some repetitive tasks, such as wax modeling, tooth insertion, milling, packing, and crafting hooks; there may be awkward postures of the upper body. Pedals were frequently used.

With regard to the presence of pollutants, certain materials produce dust (gypsum, pumice); gas is constantly used to operate the Bunsen burners; there are fumes (from welding metal alloys) and other substances (methyl methacrylate, silica, cristobalite and tridymite, chromium/cobalt/molybdenum) which, although in limited quantities, are classified as irritating, sensitizing, and carcinogenic. In short, pollutants are present even though in minor quantities in the form of dust, smoke or steam; at times the operations are not performed under the extractor hood.

With regard to the use of tools and machinery, acidic substances were replaced, in our sample laboratory, with ultrasound equipment consisting of a generator that produces acoustic shock energy capable of detaching impurities even in cavities that are difficult to reach manually. Certain tools and equipment may cause accidents even though they are kept in good repair: the debris produced by cutters and grinders may cause injury, pliers and spatulas may cause abrasions, Bunsen burners may cause burns from contact with the flame.

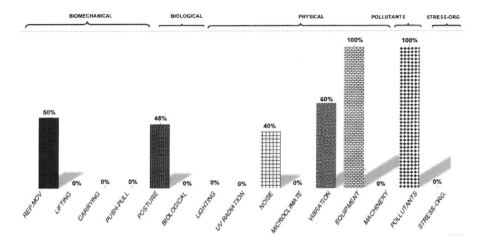

FIGURE 11.10 Results of the first initial assessment of discomfort and hazards with the pre-mapping work sheet: Emerging issues and priorities.

As far as *physical agents* are concerned, certain tools transmit vibrations to the hand and arm (e.g. plaster vibrator and polisher). Some equipment is also noisy (e.g. extractor hood, mallet for divesting molds) which, however, do not prevent the operators from talking to each other.

No lighting issues were detected, nor microclimate or UV radiation problems.

The pre-mapping model provides an overview of the risk descriptors through the observation of the tasks. The results of the pre-mapping analysis (Figure 11.10) lead us to focus on the risks deriving from the equipment but also the risk caused by the misuse of substances.

11.3.5 CONCLUSIONS AND REMARKS REGARDING THE RESULTS

This study certainly does not claim to be exhaustive in describing all the tasks that may be performed in all types of dental laboratories.

Since the instruments used in most (Italian) laboratories in this sector are largely manual, the assessment must focus on simple equipment and machinery rather than on the complexity of larger facilities.

The craftsmanship displayed so extensively in the sector also determined its fragmentation, making it often difficult to approach the assessment process; hence the need for simple software tools with which to instantly gauge the hazards present in the working environment of the dental laboratory.

This is why pre-mapping models for hazard analysis were utilized: Certain activities were found to involve repetitive tasks; chemical–physical pollutants and problems arising from the use of equipment were detected. As a result, a more in-depth analysis should be carried out by evaluating and measuring the potential risks highlighted in this study.

Without going so far as to suggest the potential replacement of the materials and products used and bearing in mind the routine use of personal protective equipment (gloves, masks, goggles), the simple measures indicated below could improve working conditions in our sample laboratory going forward.

Fume extractor systems were found to be effective for milling operations but not when using materials that produce dust (gypsum) and mixing resins that use methyl methacrylate. A simple solution could be to install a portable extractor fan along the line, where powders and dust-producing substances are used and placing it as close as possible to the point of emission.

Noise and vibrations could also be reduced through constant monitoring and regular equipment maintenance, in addition to possibly redesigning the workstations and installing damper plates.

In conclusion, this study aims to be a starting point and reference framework for employers in a sector that is still poorly investigated; it might, however, also be useful to occupational safety and health specialists including physicians responsible for defining protocols designed to ensure effective health surveillance.

11.4 ANALYSIS OF THE SOURCES OF RISK AND BIOMECHANICAL OVERLOAD AMONG BAR ATTENDANTS OR BARISTI

Sergio Ardissone
Ergonomics of Posture and Movements International Ergonomics School (EPM-IES)

11.4.1 INTRODUCTION

Throughout history, humans have had to deal with the problem of finding enough to eat and drink. As time went by, people eventually began distributing and selling the food and beverages they most needed and enjoyed. Initially, traders travelled from place to place, but at a certain point, establishments were set up where the products of the earth were transformed into appetizing foods but, above all, where beverages were sold that no longer merely quenched people's thirst, but also "lifted the mood and boosted courage". Over the centuries, these refreshment points became increasingly specialized, not only for serving food and drinks but as places where people could congregate and socialize. In Italy, the foodservice and hospitality sector has grown significantly over recent decades, expanding throughout the length and breadth of the country, with countless small and artisanal businesses popping up, and larger establishments located especially along major rail and road arteries. According to late 2015 statistics (FIEPET, 2015), Italy had some 363,000 such businesses, of which 46% bars, with 170,000 employees, and 54% restaurants, with 193,000 employees. Some 69.50% of Italian cafes and restaurants (252,308) are located in the northern and central regions of the country, followed by the southern regions, Sicily and Sardinia, with 110,977 establishments (30.50% of the total), as can be seen in Table 11.4.

On average, there are six businesses per thousand inhabitants, of which 2.8 bars and 3.2 restaurants.

TABLE 11.4

Distribution of Italian Bars and Restaurants (Number) Broken Down by Geographical Areas

	Cafe	Restaurants	Total
North Central Italy	119.970	132.338	252.308
South Italy and Islands	49.627	61.350	110.977
Italy	**169.597**	**193.688**	**363.285**

Source: FIEPET (2015).

The safety issues and health risks associated with these businesses are often underestimated, leading to the possibility of workplace accidents and occupational diseases and disorders affecting employees. According to 2018 data provided by INAIL, in the period 2013–2017 the trend in the hotel, bar and foodservice sector was largely stable (INAIL, 2018). There were 20,583 work-related accidents in 2013, and 19,430 in 2017. The most common causes include slips, sudden movements and loss of control of tools and sharp objects, which mainly cause injuries to the hands, spine and lower limbs. The occupation with the highest accident rate is cooks, accounting for 22% of the total, followed by waiters (21%), kitchen workers (13%), barmen (7%) and pizza makers (4%).

The most frequently reported occupational health problems are skin diseases, tendinitis, intervertebral disc diseases, carpal tunnel syndrome and other peripheral neuropathies.

11.4.2 THE TECHNOLOGICAL CYCLE (ARDISSONE, 2011)

The job of the bar attendant involves various tasks, the number of which varies according to the size of the establishment and the professionalism required. This study looked into the very complex environment of cafes at service stations located on major motorways. The relentless flow of large numbers of customers calls for staff to handle a wide variety of tasks. The pace (especially in peak hours) is particularly high: the work is performed over various shifts (morning – afternoon – night) and cover the entire day; night shifts seem particularly problematic.

The tasks can be divided into four groups (Figure 11.11):

- *Tasks at the counter* (making coffee, serving drinks by the glass, dispensing beverages on tap, cash sales, cash transactions with the sale of cigarettes, sandwiches, cakes and croissants);
- *Tasks in the kitchen* (preparing sandwiches and rolls);
- *Washing and cleaning* (washing glasses, cups and saucers, crockery, etc., washing pots and pans in the kitchen, cleaning the counter, cleaning tables and cleaning floors);
- *Stock management* (stacking shelves with beverages, storing raw materials, etc.).

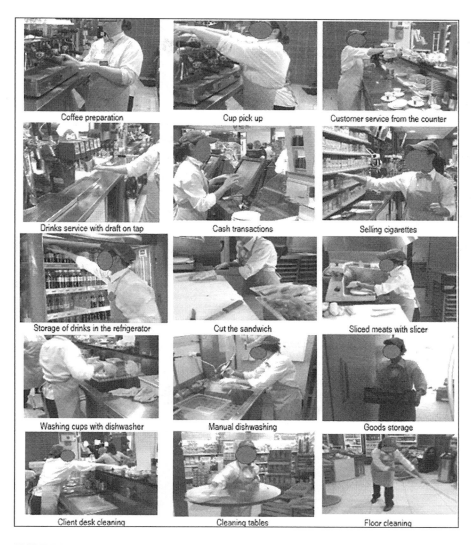

FIGURE 11.11   Illustrations of the main tasks of the bar attendant.

11.4.2.1   Tasks at the Counter

These tasks involve dealing directly with patrons and, at particular times of the day or night, the work of serving an unrelenting flow of customers is very fast paced. The work requires the bar attendant to move along the length of the counter and use worktops placed at different heights, with possible problems arising due to non-ergonomic design. Table 11.5 shows the main tasks performed by the bar attendant or barista at the counter.

TABLE 11.5

Analytical Description of the Main Tasks Performed by the Bar Attendant at the Counter and the Main Cleaning and Washing Tasks

Main tasks related to counter operations
Coffee preparation
Beverage service by the glass
Beverage service on tap
Cash transactions
Cash transactions with cigarette sales
Sandwiches, sweets, brioches service
Main tasks concerning cleaning and washing operations
Dishwashing with dishwasher
Manual dishwashing
Counter cleaning
Cleaning tables
Floor cleaning

11.4.2.2   Tasks in the Kitchen

There is almost always a kitchen on the premises, where different types of food are prepared (sandwiches, hot croissants, ready-made meals, etc.). The equipment and appliances are not always efficient and safe, and their positioning is sometimes ergonomically incorrect.

Preparation of sandwiches, rolls, etc. After preparing all the ingredients on the work surface, the operator slices the loaf or rolls with a knife and fills them; the most popular ingredients are cold cut; often, the operator has a slicer at his or her disposal (in most cases operated manually). Once prepared, the sandwiches and rolls are loaded on a platter or tray and placed in a display case. The right shoulder can often be in an awkward position.

11.4.2.3   Cleaning and Washing

These seemingly simple tasks take up much of the bar attendant's shift. Table 11.5 lists the main tasks involved in cleaning and washing.

11.4.2.4   Stock Management

Stock needs taking care of several times a day and the work consists mainly in manually transporting loads from the storeroom to the point of sale; the worker uses force to lift, carry, push, pull or otherwise move objects.

Storing raw materials. Incoming raw materials are normally deposited by external delivery firms in a pre-established point adjacent to the premises: it is the duty of the staff to transport the packages (boxes, crates, parcels) to the storeroom. Some of the loads weigh more than 3 kg and as much as 10–12 kg. The use of considerable force and the awkward postures of the hands throughout almost the entire cycle make this task one of the most taxing in terms of biomechanical overload of the upper limbs.

Stocking beverages on shelves. Beverages, whether in bottles or cans, are handled manually in cartons or boxes that always weigh more than 3 kg. The operator picks up the loads from the storeroom and carries them over sometimes quite long distances to the premises; when the package is opened, he or she places the individual bottle or can on the various shelves of the display units. As for the previous task, considerable lifting force is used, and the shoulder is in an awkward posture.

11.4.3 DEFINITION OF THE HOMOGENEOUS GROUP

At the establishment studied here, the work is organized in three shifts: morning (6 am–2 pm), afternoon (2 pm–10 pm) and night (10 pm–6 am).

At around the middle of the shift there is a 20-minute meal break, included in the working hours (and thus paid). There are another two unofficial 10-minute breaks.

There was a total of 16 employees at the establishment examined here, with 3–4 people working the morning shift, 2–3 the afternoon shift and only 1 person on the night shift. The workers are randomly assigned to the various weekly shifts.

Since all the employees carry out all the tasks, only one homogeneous group was identified and analyzed.

11.4.4 RESULTS OF PRELIMINARY STUDIES: ANALYSIS OF DISCOMFORT AND HAZARDS USING THE PRE-MAPPING WORK SHEET

The pre-mapping work sheet described in previous chapters was applied to bar attendants. The results are depicted in the graph in Figure 11.12.

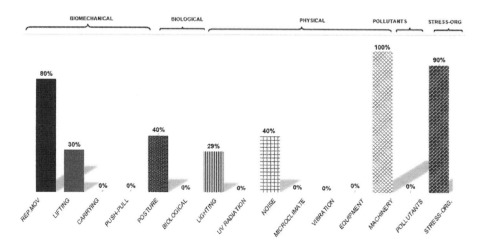

FIGURE 11.12 The main risk factors for the bar attendant as detected using the pre-mapping work sheet.

The results show that there are risks for the health and safety of workers in the technological cycle, especially biomechanical, organizational and physical risks. In order of importance, the following forms of discomfort or exposure hazards are present:

- Risk due to the presence of equipment that can cause cuts, scratches or burns.
- Risk due to organizational factors, since the employees work several shifts, even at night, when there only one operator is on duty; moreover, at peak times (breakfast, lunch, weekends, public holidays), crowds can generate a particularly high work pace.
- The risk of repetitive movements is present in virtually all tasks.
- Workers are at risk for awkward postures when carrying out their tasks. They must stand for most of the shift and there is moderate bending of the trunk.
- Noise due to crowds of customers on the premises causes discomfort during peak times.
- Stock management tasks place workers at risk due to lifting loads weighing more than 3 kg.

11.4.5   CONCLUSIONS

The final brief indications suggest the need for a more in-depth evaluation of the biomechanical risks which, after applying albeit the simplified risk analysis models, were found to be quite significantly present. The study also shows that, in the sector in question and considering what was observed in the specific business, there are in fact physical hazards due mainly to the presence of the machines and equipment typically used in the sector and often poorly maintained. The effectiveness of the methodology employed in this study is further demonstrated by the detection of organizational risks, which may be a significant source of stress and are probably responsible for mental and physical disorders and diseases among employees.

The adoption of efficient operating procedures in order to change how tasks are performed (e.g. using both hands, eliminating unnecessary actions, correcting awkward postures) and a thorough study of the ergonomic design of the workstations, together with appropriate information, education and training, would significantly reduce the risk of biomechanical overload. Periodical inspections and maintenance of the machines used by bar attendants would also go a long way towards reducing workplace accidents and injuries.

12 Pre-mapping in an Agricultural Setting

Presentation of a Specific ERGOCHECK Model

Daniela Colombini and Enrico Occhipinti
Ergonomics of Posture and Movements
International Ergonomics School (EPM-IES)

CONTENTS

12.1   FOREWORD

Agriculture is by far the world's largest industry. It is estimated that 40% of today's working population – some 2.6 billion people – are farmers. Agriculture is one of the most hazardous occupations in both emerging and highly developed economies.

The fact that farm workers often carry out numerous activities at different days and/or months of the year makes risk assessments extremely complex. This is why it is crucial to conduct an in-depth preliminary analysis on how agricultural work is organized.

Preliminary studies must be carried out even before hazards and work-related issues are pre-mapped using ERGOCHECK. The purpose is to report exposure which, in agricultural settings, tends to vary in duration at different times of the year and, therefore, to be associated with different risk factors. Without this information, risk levels would clearly be regarded as identical regardless of whether workers are exposed to full-time, part-time or seasonal work.

Given the complexity of organizational studies in agriculture, a simple yet specialized digital tool has been developed to help operators pre-map the discomfort and dangers involved in farm work. This tool is illustrated over the next few pages.

Two models are available:

- **EPMIES-agriERGOCHECKprecultivoENG:** The first is a *universal cultivation model of approach,* already broken down into macro-phases and tasks, that can be adapted to many crops and is the easier of the two to use; this is the model used in all the examples below.
- **EPMIES-multiannoERGOCHECKpremapENG:** The second version uses the same calculation models but the macro-phases and tasks are blank. It may be used not only in agriculture but also other industries in which many different tasks are performed at different times throughout the year (such as building construction).

12.2   GENERAL PRE-MAPPING MODEL FOR AGRICULTURE: A FACILITATED ORGANIZATIONAL ANALYSIS

The general organizational process underlying a pre-mapping analysis, or an actual exposure risk assessment, requires a step-by-step approach. First of all, the various tasks involved in the crop growing or cultivation process must be identified from the qualitative and quantitative standpoint. Next, the distribution of tasks throughout the year is analyzed. Lastly, the tasks are matched to the workers and the workers are divided into homogeneous groups. This complex study, including the pre-mapping part, is illustrated over the coming pages.

12.2.1   PHASE 1: IDENTIFICATION OF TASKS INVOLVED IN CULTIVATION

As it is so inherently difficult to identify macro-phases, phases and tasks in the crop growing or cultivation process (Colombini and Occhipinti 2014, 2017), a kind of *universal cultivation approach* has been developed that will enable even beginners

Main pre-defined tasks	
PREPARATION AND TREATMENT OF SOIL, MECHANICAL WEEDING	with tractor with animals with manual tools manual carrying (weight up to max. 3 kg) manual carrying (weight 3 kg) with manual tool and pulling/pushing other activities, without tools, with repetitive movements of the upper limbs (without lifting up to max.3 kg) other activities, without tools, with repetitive movements of the upper limbs (with lifting up to max.3 kg)
DISINFECTION, DISINFESTATION, FERTILIZING, CHEMICAL WEEDING	with tractor manual with machinery manual with tools with manual tools and pulling/pushing other activities, without tools, with repetitive movements of the upper limbs (without lifting, up to max.3 kg) other activities, without tools, with repetitive movements of the upper limbs (with lifting, up to max 3 kg)
PLANTING	automatic with tractor semi-automatic with tools and / or machinery manual with manual tool (product weight up to max. 3 kg) manual without tools (product weight up to max. 3 kg) manual with manual tool (product weight over 3 kg) manual without tools (product weight over 3 kg) manual carrying (product weight up to max. 3 kg) manual carrying (product weight above 3 kg) with manual tool and pulling/pushing other activities, without tools, with repetitive movements of the upper limbs (without lifting, up to max. 3 kg) other activities, without tools, with repetitive movements of the upper limbs (with lifting, up to max. 3 kg)
INTERMEDIATE FARM WORK (PRUNING, BINDING, THINNING, ETC.)	pruning with manual tools pruning with pneumatic / electric tools pruning with chainsaws manual pruning without tools manual carrying (weight up to max. 3 kg) manual carrying (weight 3 kg) with manual tool and pulling/ pushing other activities, without tools, with repetitive movements of the upper limbs (without lifting, up to max. 3 kg) other activities, without tools, with repetitive movements of the upper limbs (with lifting, up to max. 3 kg)
HARVESTING OF CROPS	automatic with tractor semi-automatic with tools and / or machinery manual with manual tool manual with pneumatic / electric tools manual with chainsaw manual with animal manual without tools manual carrying (weight up to max. 3 kg) manual carrying (weight 3 kg) with manual tool and pulling/pushing other activities, without tools, with repetitive movements of the upper limbs (without lifting, up to max. 3 kg) other activities, without tools, with repetitive movements of the upper limbs (with lifting up to max. 3 kg)

FIGURE 12.1 Principal tasks characterizing a generic cultivation activity.

to conduct a preliminary organizational analysis in an agricultural setting. It consists of macro-phases (soil preparation, treatment, disinfection and fertilization, planting, intermediate processes and harvesting) that include a certain number of typical tasks broken down by type, technique and/or the tool(s) used or load(s) handled (Figure 12.1).

12.2.2 PHASE 2: IDENTIFICATION OF A HOMOGENEOUS GROUP

The software mentioned above requires the completion of an organizational analysis that is presented on page 1 (1-ORGANIZATION) and begins with the identification of homogeneous groups.

The next step is to assign tasks to individual workers or groups of workers exposed to the same risk, i.e. to identify homogeneous groups. For each type of crop, tasks will be assigned to different groups of workers. When tasks of the same type and duration are assigned to the same group of workers, we may speak of a *homogeneous group in terms of risk exposure*. A homogeneous group may sometimes be comprised of one person, if no other workers perform the same task (from the qualitative and quantitative standpoint).

For instance, typically, a single group of workers may be assigned the job of actually growing a certain crop (tasks may include pruning, harvesting, etc.), while other workers prepare and disinfect the soil, apply fertilizers and so on.

The **EPMIES-agriERGOCHECKprecultivoENG** software should be used creating a file for each homogeneous group assigned to cultivating one or more crops during the year: each homogeneous group thus has a separate file.

Having opened the *pre-defined universal cultivation* document, an "X" is placed in the appropriate column to activate the tasks performed by the homogeneous group, for subsequent analytical quantification. The various tasks performed during different months of the year are thus recorded qualitatively and quantitatively (in percentages). The sum of the percentages indicated for each month must always add up to 100%. The percentages need not be perfectly accurate; they only describe the proportion of time spent each month performing a certain task.

Figure 12.2 shows an example of a form filled out for a homogeneous group of full-time workers at a large farm that grows top-quality wine grapes. This homogeneous group of about ten male workers performs many tasks that are variously distributed throughout the year.

To report the quantitative data required to define exposure durations, for each month, it is necessary to enter the number of hours worked by each worker. It is important to remember that as the group is homogeneous, all the members of the group work the same number of hours.

Figure 12.2 also shows that the total number of hours worked per month may vary considerably.

12.2.3   Phase 3: Definition of DURATION MULTIPLIERS for Adjusting Risk Scores Based on Their Specific Duration

The software then converts the total number of hours worked per month into percentages with respect to a constant 160 hours/month, which corresponds to 8 working hours per day, 5 days a week, 4 weeks a month (Colombini and Occhipinti 2014, 2017). Therefore, if the percentage is 100% that means that the number of hours worked that month is the same as the constant; if the percentage is higher or lower, it means that exposure to work-related risk is proportionally greater or lesser: deviations from the exposure constants become the basic criteria for calculating variations in risk levels (or priorities) as a function of changes in exposure duration.

Figure 12.3a shows the percentage of hours worked per month (by homogeneous group 1 in the example depicted in Figure 12.2), obtained by dividing the number of hours/worker by a constant 160 hours/month.

It is now possible to assign these duration percentages, on a month by month basis, to certain risk factors where the total number of hours worked coincides with the duration of exposure to that particular risk factor: repetitive movements, awkward postures, lighting, micro-climate, UV radiation from outdoor work, and

Notes	Main pre-defined tasks	SIGN WITH "X" THE ACTIVE TASKS	HOURS WORKED PER MONTH PER WORKER JAN 0	FEB 160	MAR 160	APR 160	MAY 160	JUN 160	JUL 160	AUG 160	SEP 200	OCT 200	NOV 100	DEC 50
PREPARATION AND TREATMENT OF SOIL, MECHANICAL WEEDING	with tractor					5%	5%							30%
	with animals													10%
	with manual tools	X		10%					10%					20%
	manual carrying (weight up to max. 3 kg)				20%	30%	5%		5%				5%	
	manual carrying (weight 3 kg)													
	with manual tool and pulling/pushing													
	other activities, without tools, with repetitive movements of the upper limbs (without lifting up to max.3													
	other activities, without tools, with repetitive movements of the upper limbs (with lifting up to max.3 kg)	X							2.5%					
DISINFECTION, DISINFESTATION, FERTILIZING, CHEMICAL WEEDING	with tractor													
	manual with machinery								10%					
	manual with tools			10%										
	with manual tools and pulling/pushing													
	other activities, without tools, with repetitive movements of the upper limbs (without lifting up to max.3								2.5%					
	other activities, without tools, with repetitive movements of the upper limbs (with lifting up to max.3 kg)	X							2.5%					10%
PLANTING	automatic with tractor													
	semi-automatic with tools and / or machinery													
	manual with manual tool (product weight up to max. 3 kg)			30%		5%	5%							
	manual without tools (product weight up to max 3 kg)	X				5%	5%		2.5%		10%	10%		
	manual with manual tool (product weight over 3 kg)				10%	10%	10%							
	manual carrying (product weight up to max. 3 kg)	X			10%	10%	10%							
	manual carrying (product weight above 3 kg)			10%	10%	10%								
	with manual tool and pulling/pushing			10%										
	other activities, without tools, with repetitive movements of the upper limbs (without lifting up to max.3	X							2.5%	10%	10%	10%		
	other activities, without tools, with repetitive movements of the upper limbs (with lifting up to max.3 kg)	X						30%	75%	40%				
INTERMEDIATE FARM WORK (PRUNING, BINDING, THINNING, ETC.)	pruning with manual tools				5%	5%	5%						5%	
	pruning with pneumatic / electric tools													
	pruning with chainsaws													
	manual pruning without tools													
	manual carrying (weight up to max 3 kg)					5%	5%			10%				
	manual carrying (weight 3 kg)				30%			5%						
	with manual tool and pulling/pushing													
	other activities, without tools, with repetitive movements of the upper limbs (without lifting up to max.3	X							10%	10%	10%	60%		
	other activities, without tools, with repetitive movements of the upper limbs (with lifting up to max.3 kg)	X							10%	10%	10%			
HARVESTING OF CROPS	automatic with tractor					45%								
	semi-automatic with tools and / or machinery											5%		
	manual with manual tool									10%	10%	5%		
	manual with pneumatic / electric tools			30%		5%	5%		70%	70%	80%	70%		
	manual with chainsaw													
	manual with animal													
	manual without tools	X		30%	5%			5%					10%	10%
	manual carrying (weight up to max. 3 kg)	X		10%							10%	10%	10%	
	manual carrying (weight 3 kg)													
	with manual tool and pulling/pushing	X						5%						
	other activities, without tools, with repetitive movements of the upper limbs (without lifting up to max.3	X											10%	10%
	other activities, without tools, with repetitive movements of the upper limbs (with lifting up to max.3 kg)	X											10%	10%
	THE SUM TOTAL PER MONTH MUST ALWAYS ADD UP TO 100%		0%	100%	100%	100%	100%	100%	100%	100%	100%	100%	100%	100%

FIGURE 12.2 Identification in the *pre-defined universal cultivation* form of tasks performed by the homogeneous group (activated by entering an "X"). Qualitative and quantitative distribution (in percentages) of the various tasks performed in the different months of the year. The sum of the percentages indicated for each month must add up to 100%.

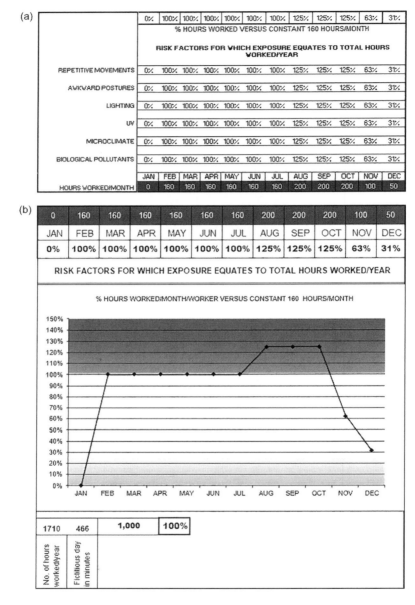

FIGURE 12.3 (a) Percentage of hours worked per month (by the homogeneous group in the example), obtained by dividing the number of hours/worker by the constant 160 hours/month. These percentages can now be assigned, on a month by month basis, to certain risk factors where the total number of hours worked coincides with the duration of exposure to that particular risk factor. (b) Graph plotting the monthly distribution of tasks with durations indicated in percentages versus a constant 160 hours/month. Lines in the red area mean that the constant is exceeded. Calculation of the *fictitious working day* that converts the total duration of hours worked/year into a single day, by comparing with the constants.

biological pollutants are almost always present and inherently linked to farm work (Figure 12.3).

Figure 12.3b visually plots the monthly distribution of work in percentages versus the constant 160 hours/month. The curves in the red area indicate levels above the constant; the number of hours worked per month is also not evenly distributed – it rises during the harvest season.

The figures below the graph indicate the duration in hours worked on the *fictitious working day*; this calculation converts the total duration of hours worked/year into a single day, by comparing the constants. In the calculation, 100% means that the year is equivalent to a fictitious 8-hour day (multiplier 1 for the DURATION FACTOR, as per the Occupational Repetitive Action, OCRA checklist method). The number of hours worked per year in the example amounts to 1,736 (which is very close to the constant 1,760 hours/year). Dividing this figure by 220 working days/year and multiplying the result by 60 obtains the number of minutes in the fictitious working day representing the time worked in the year: 473 minutes in this example.

Based on the data shown in Table 12.1 (illustrating the DURATION MULTIPLIERS used to adjust the risk indexes as a function of task duration, as per the OCRA checklist), it can be seen that the Multiplier corresponding to 473 minutes is equal to 1, therefore, the risk calculated for this situation is unchanged: the *fictitious day* has a duration of 421–480 minutes.

If one considers tasks that involve lifting loads weighing 3 kg or more, it is essential to examine the actual duration of such tasks throughout the year, which will undoubtedly be lower than the duration attributed to the aforementioned potential risk factors (because not all the tasks listed involve manual load lifting). This critical data is easy to obtain (in order to avoid overestimating exposure) by placing an "X" in the form against tasks featuring the characteristics indicated here: the hours of exposure automatically appear for each individual task along with the total for each

---

TABLE 12.1

DURATION MULTIPLIERS for Adjusting Risk Indexes (or Priority Levels) as a Function of Task Duration (Colombini & Occhipinti, 2017; 2019)

DURATION MULTIPLIERS Used for the OCRA Checklist

Net Time (min.)	DURATION MULTIPLIER	Net Time (min.)	DURATION MULTIPLIER
0–1.86	0.007	241–300	0.85
1.87–3.74	0.018	301–360	0.925
3.75–7.4	0.05	361–421	0.95
7.5–14.99	0.1	421–480	1
15–29.99	0.2	481–539	1.2
30–59.99	0.35	540–599	1.5
60–120	0.5	600–659	2
121–180	0.65	660–719	2.8
181–240	0.75	720	4

month. The estimated percentages are then calculated with respect to the constant 160 hours/month (Figure 12.4).

If the software **EPMIES-agriERGOCHECKprecultivoENG** *with pre-defined tasks for universal cultivation* is used, the tasks entailing manual lifting are already activated, but can be modified if necessary.

Figures 12.5–12.7 show the results of the search for exposure duration data for the remaining risk factors. Figure 12.5 shows the risk factors for *manually carrying* and *pushing/pulling* (the names of the pre-entered tasks emphasize the existence of these jobs): here too, when such tasks are present, they appear already activated in the software with an "X" in the appropriate place (as described for Figure 12.4).

Figure 12.6 shows the risk factors for *noise* and *vibrations from vibrating tools.* The attribution of possible risk due to noise is applied to all tasks involving the use of vibrating tools, as well as for tasks that involve driving farm vehicles.

Lastly, Figure 12.7 shows the risk factors associated with the use of *inadequate equipment and machinery* and exposure to *whole-body vibrations,* again with a view to calculating the actual duration of exposure.

As described for Figure 12.3b, the graphs in Figures 12.8 and 12.9 depict the distribution of working hours in percentages for the various risk factors: it is easy to see how the potential duration of exposure will differ considerably in relation to the various risk factors and months of the year.

For each risk factor, we now have an estimated duration in the fictitious working day (representative of the exposure year), and with it the relative DURATION MULTIPLIER and its value in percentages.

This value is of the utmost importance because it is used to modify the weight of each individual risk factor versus its actual duration: these values are necessary for determining priorities. The classic ERGOCHECK program for each risk factor, based on the replies provided by the homogeneous group, calculates a score. This score will now be modified (increased, decreased or even left unchanged) with respect to the DURATION MULTIPLIER: if it remains at 100% no changes will be made; if it is below 100% the weight associated with that risk factor will decrease proportionally; the opposite will be the case if it is above 100%. It is worth remembering that the value is 100% when the duration of exposure is equal to the pre-defined exposure constants, i.e. 160 working hours/month, 11 months/year, 1,760 working hours/year.

EPMIES-agriERGOCHECKprecultivoENG automatically calculates the DURATION MULTIPLIER and applies it to the various risk factors: obviously this is only possible if the data entered for organizational analysis in Work Sheet 1 indicates the number of hours worked/month and the duration in percentages of the various tasks performed by the homogeneous group each month.

	Activity		
PREPARATION AND TREATMENT OF SOIL, MECHANICAL WEEDING	with tractor		
	with animals		
	with manual tools		
	manual carrying (weight up to max 3 kg)	X	
	manual carrying (weight 3 kg)	X	
	with manual tool and pulling/pushing		
	other activities, without tools, with repetitive movements of the upper limbs (without lifting up to max 3		
	other activities, without tools, with repetitive movements of the upper limbs (with lifting up to max 3 kg)	X	
DISINFECTION, DISINFESTATION, FERTILIZING, CHEMICAL WEEDING	with tractor		
	manual with machinery		
	manual with tools		
	with manual tools and pulling/pushing		
	other activities, without tools, with repetitive movements of the upper limbs (without lifting up to max.3		
	other activities, without tools, with repetitive movements of the upper limbs (with lifting up to max 3 kg)	X	
PLANTING	automatic with tractor		
	semi-automatic with tools and / or machinery		
	manual with manual tool (product weight up to max. 3 kg)		
	manual without tools (product weight up to max. 3 kg)	X	
	manual without tools (product weight over 3 kg)	X	
	manual carrying (product weight up to max. 3 kg)		
	manual carrying (product weight above 3 kg)	X	
	with manual tool and pulling/pushing		
	other activities, without tools, with repetitive movements of the upper limbs (without lifting up to max. 3		
	other activities, without tools, with repetitive movements of the upper limbs (with lifting up to max 3 kg)	X	
INTERMEDIATE FARM WORK (PRUNING, BINDING, THINNING ETC)	pruning with manual tools		
	pruning with pneumatic / electric tools		
	pruning with chainsaws		
	manual pruning without tools	X	
	manual carrying (weight up to max. 3 kg)		
	manual carrying (weight 3 kg)	X	
	with manual tool and pulling/ pushing		
	other activities, without tools, with repetitive movements of the upper limbs (without lifting up to max 3		
	other activities, without tools, with repetitive movements of the upper limbs (with lifting up to max 3 kg)	X	
HARVESTING OF CROPS	automatic with tractor		
	semi-automatic with tools and / or machinery		
	manual with manual tool	X	
	manual with pneumatic / electric tools		
	manual with chainsaw		
	manual with animal		
	manual without tools		
	manual carrying (weight up to max. 3 kg)	X	
	manual carrying (weight 3 kg)		
	with manual tool and pulling/pushing		
	other activities, without tools, with repetitive movements of the upper limbs (without lifting up to max 3	X	
	other activities, without tools, with repetitive movements of the upper limbs (with lifting up to max 3 kg)	X	

THE SUM TOTAL PER MONTH MUST ALWAYS ADD UP TO 100%

DURATION OF TASKS THAT INVOLVE LOAD HANDLING

	JAN	FEB	MAR	APR	MAY	JUN	JUL	AUG	SEP	OCT	NOV	DEC
	0	64	80	80	40	8	8	28	0	0	20	0
	0%	40%	50%	50%	25%	5%	5%	18%	0%	0%	13%	0%

FIGURE 12.4 Calculation of the number of hours worked/year only for tasks that involve the manual lifting of loads weighing equal to or more than 3 kg. Sum of the hours/month and calculation of percentages versus the constant 160 hours/month.

		DURATION OF TASKS THAT INVOLVE CARRYING												DURATION OF TASKS THAT INVOLVE PUSHING/PULLING											

with tractor
with animals
with manual tools
manual carrying (weight up to max. 3 kg)
with manual tool and pulling/pushing
other activities, without tools, with repetitive movements of the upper limbs (without lifting up to max. 3 kg)
other activities, without tools, with repetitive movements of the upper limbs (with lifting up to max. 3 kg)

with tractor
manual with machinery
manual with tools
with manual tools and pulling/pushing
other activities, without tools, with repetitive movements of the upper limbs (without lifting up to max. 3 kg)
other activities, without tools, with repetitive movements of the upper limbs (with lifting up to max. 3 kg)

automatic with tractor
semi-automatic with tools and / or machinery
manual with manual tool (product weight up to max. 3 kg)
manual without tools (product weight up to max. 3 kg)
manual with manual tool (product weight over 3 kg)
manual without tools (product weight over 3 kg)
manual carrying (product weight up to max. 3 kg)
manual carrying (product weight above 3 kg)
with manual tool and pulling/pushing
other activities, without tools, with repetitive movements of the upper limbs (without lifting up to max. 3 kg)
other activities, without tools, with repetitive movements of the upper limbs (with lifting up to max. 3 kg)

pruning with manual tools
pruning with pneumatic / electric tools
pruning with chainsaws
manual pruning without tools
manual carrying (weight up to max. 3 kg)
manual carrying (weight 3 kg)
with manual tool and pulling/ pushing
other activities, without tools, with repetitive movements of the upper limbs (without lifting up to max. 3 kg)
other activities, without tools, with repetitive movements of the upper limbs (with lifting up to max. 3 kg)

automatic with tractor
semi-automatic with tools and / or machinery
manual with manual tool
manual with pneumatic / electric tools
manual with chainsaw
manual with animal
manual without tools
manual carrying (weight up to max. 3 kg)
manual carrying (weight 3 kg)
with manual tool and pulling/pushing
other activities, without tools, with repetitive movements of the upper limbs (without lifting up to max. 3 kg)
other activities, without tools, with repetitive movements of the upper limbs (with lifting up to max. 3 kg)

THE SUM TOTAL PER MONTH MUST ALWAYS ADD UP TO 100%

	JA	FE	MA	AP	MA	JUN	JUL	AU	SE	OC	NO	DE
CARRYING	0	16	64	64	24	0	28	0	0	0	20	16
PUSHING/PULLING	0	48	32	56	8	0	4	0	20	0	5	20

FIGURE 12.5 Calculation of the number of hours worked/year only for tasks that involve the manual carrying and pushing/pulling of loads. Sum of the hours/month and calculation of percentages versus the constant 160 hours/month.

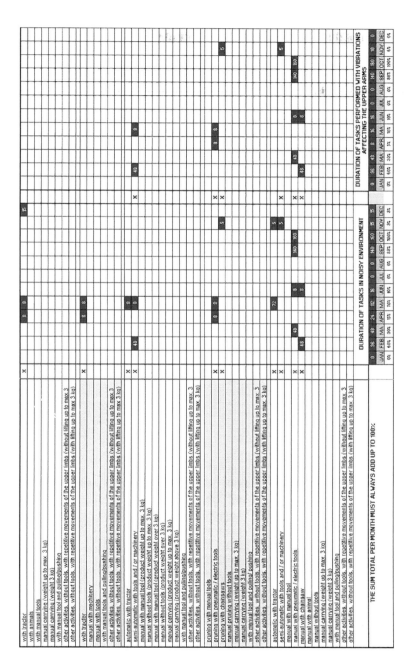

FIGURE 12.6 Calculation of the number of hours worked/year only for tasks that involve noise and upper limb vibrations. Sum of the hours/month and calculation of percentages versus the constant 160 hours/month.

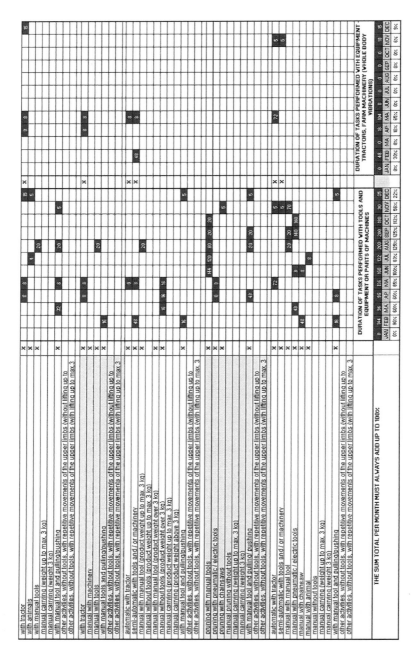

FIGURE 12.7 Calculation of the number of hours worked/year only for tasks that involve the use of tools, machinery and whole-body vibrations. Sum of the hours/month and calculation of percentages versus the constant 160 hours/month.

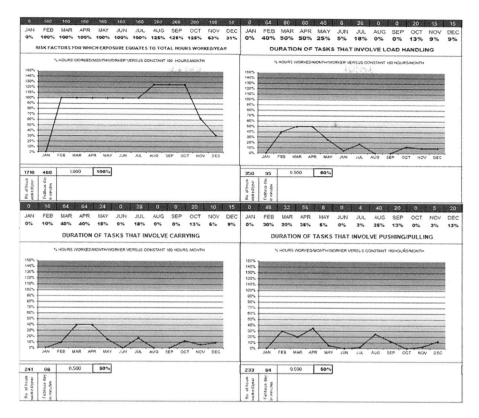

FIGURE 12.8 Distribution of the percentages of hours worked/month versus the constant 160 hours/month, for the total number of hours worked/year and for the following risk factors: manual load lifting, manual load carrying and pushing/pulling. Estimated duration of the corresponding *fictitious days* (or representative day of the year) and calculation of the DURATION MULTIPLIER and corresponding level in %.

12.3 SIMILARITIES AND DIFFERENCES BETWEEN EPMIES AGRI ERGOCHECK PRECULTIVO ENG AND THE CLASSIC ERGOCHECK MODEL

12.3.1 RESULTS OF THE FIRST SECTION REGARDING *KEY-ENTERS* FOR BIOMECHANICAL OVERLOAD AND *KEY-QUESTIONS* REGARDING OTHER RISK FACTORS

Having entered all the necessary organizational data (i.e. tasks and task durations for each month of the year) into the first work sheet of the **EPMIES-agriERGOCHECKprecultivoENG** program, and automatically generated the specific DURATION MULTIPLIERS for each risk factor, it is now possible to fill in the various sections as per the classic ERGOCHECK model described in previous

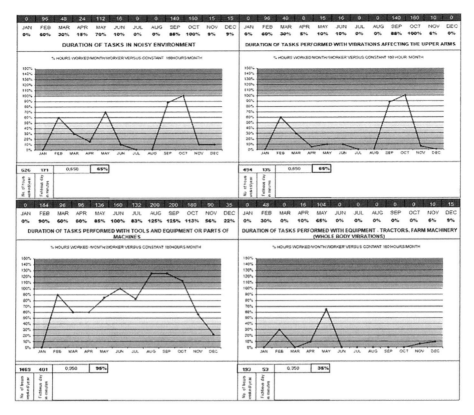

FIGURE 12.9 Distribution of the percentage of hours worked/month versus the constant 160 hours/month, for the following risk factors: noise, upper limb vibrations, inadequate equipment and machinery, whole-body vibrations. Estimated duration of the corresponding *fictitious days* (or representative day of the year) and calculation of the DURATION MULTIPLIER and corresponding level in %.

chapters. Each risk factor present appears automatically in percentage terms per month, and the DURATION MULTIPLIERS automatically adjust the risk scores for the various factors based on their actual duration.

Let's take the example analyzed earlier and depicted in Figure 12.2 (homogeneous group 1): Figure 12.10 indicates the *key-enters* for biomechanical overload due to repetitive movements, manual load lifting, manual load carrying and pushing/pulling. The data in this section appears automatically due to the *key-enters* that were marked, and to their presence (in percentages) each month of the year. The data derives from the first work sheet indicating the relevant organizational data. It can be observed that the various risk factors are present at very different levels throughout the year.

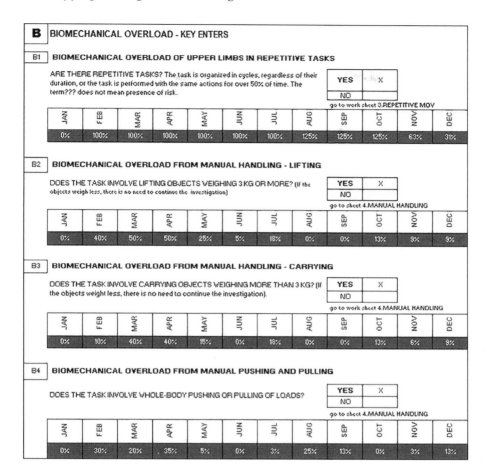

FIGURE 12.10 *Key-enters* for biomechanical overload due to repetitive movements, manual load lifting, manual carrying, pushing/pulling: qualitative and quantitative presence (in %) for each month of the year.

Figure 12.11 shows all the preliminary *key-enters* required to record the presence of awkward postures: all that needs doing is to place an "X" indicating which awkward postures are observed; a more specific work sheet is used to describe the type and duration of the main awkward postures reported by the homogeneous group.

At this point the various "sections" of the work sheet are completed for each individual risk factor, in the usual way. Figures 12.12 and 12.13 sum up the overall results. Although the DURATION MULTIPLIER cannot be seen, it nonetheless automatically modifies the risk score and consequently also the color of the "traffic light", depending on the relevant "danger level".

| B5 | BIOMECHANICAL OVERLOAD FROM AWKWARD POSTURES - TRUNK AND LOWER LIMBS |

Are there static or awkward working postures of the HEAD/NECK, TRUNK and/or UPPER AND LOWER LIMBS that are held for more than 4 seconds consecutively and repeated for a significant proportion of the working time? **YES** — X

In practice, postures are generally nto awkward (MARK "NO") when the work is performed:
- sitting with the back well supported, when there is sufficient leg room, and the subject can stand up (change position) at least every hour; **NO**

#NOME?

Examples

	NO	YES	
HEAD/NECK (neck bent back/forward/sideways, twisted)		X	
TRUNK (trunk bent forward/sideways/, back bent with no support, twisted)		X	
UPPER LIMBS (hand(s) at or above head level, elbow(s) at or above shoulder level, elbow/hand(s) behind the body, hand(s) turned with palms completely facing up or down, extreme elbow flexion-extension, wrist bent forward/back/sideways)		X	Go straight to work sheet POSTURES for trunk and lower limbs or to work sheet REPETITIVE-MOV for upper limbs
LOWER LIMBS (squatting or kneeling) position held for more than 4 seconds consecutively and repeated for a significant proportion of the working time		X	

JAN	FEB	MAR	APR	MAY	JUN	JUL	AUG	SEP	OCT	NOV	DEC
0%	100%	100%	100%	100%	100%	100%	125%	125%	125%	63%	31%

FIGURE 12.11 *Key-enters* for a preliminary definition of awkward postures.

12.3.2 RESULTS OF THE FIRST PART CONCERNING THE "QUICK ASSESSMENT" SECTIONS FOR BIOMECHANICAL OVERLOAD OF THE UPPER LIMBS

Although the *"quick assessment"* section of the work sheets is completed the same as for the classic ERGOCHECK model, all of the completed work sheets are presented here for use as exercises and for learning to use the tool later on. Figures 12.14–12.17 show the results of this initial assessment in the upper limb analysis. As the working conditions feature neither a total absence of risk (code green) nor a critical environment, the section calling for a more accurate description of the activities performed by the upper limbs is activated (Figure 12.16).

12.3.3 RESULTS OF THE SECOND PART CONCERNING THE "QUICK ASSESSMENT" SECTIONS FOR MANUAL LOAD LIFTING

Figures 12.18–12.20 show the results of this second assessment of biomechanical overload due to manual load lifting. No critical conditions emerge (but risk is not absent): the lifting is extensively reported, with loads occasionally weighing as much as 10 kg (but not exceeding critical weights).

12.3.4 RESULTS OF THE THIRD PART CONCERNING THE "QUICK ASSESSMENT" SECTIONS FOR MANUALLY CARRYING AND PUSHING/PULLING LOADS

Figure 12.21 shows the results for manual carrying: no critical conditions appear.

Figures 12.22–12.24 show the data for manual pushing and pulling and the final outcome of the overall manual load handling analysis: again, no critical conditions emerge, although there are some issues.

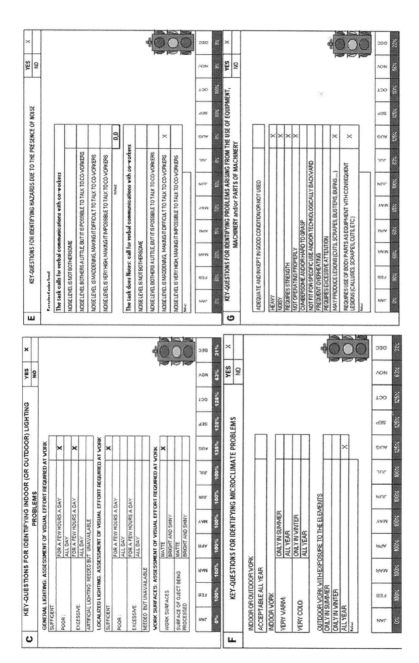

FIGURE 12.12 *Key-questions* for the study of risk factors: lighting, noise, micro-climate, use of improper/inadequate tools and machinery.

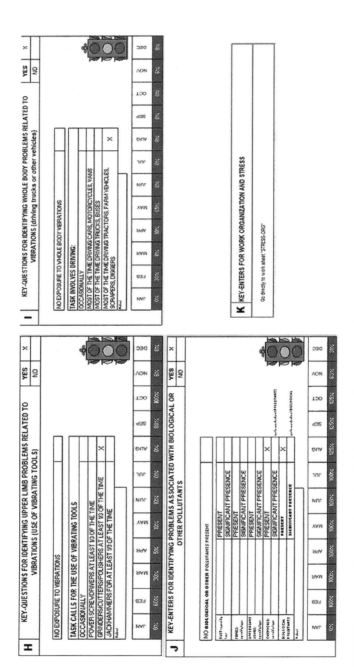

FIGURE 12.13 *Key-questions* for the study of risk factors: vibrations caused by vibrating equipment operated with the upper limbs, exposure to whole-body vibrations, or to biological/chemical pollutants, etc.

B1	BIOMECHANICAL OVERLOAD DUE TO REPETITIVE MOVEMENTS	

REPETITIVE TASK PRESENT. The task is organized in cycles, regardless of duration or the task is characterized by similar gestures performed over 50% of the time. The term does not indicate the presence of risk.	SI

Summary of repetitive work net duration on a representative average day

TOTAL shift average duration (in minutes)	480		Total repetitive working time (in minutes)	440

DESCRIPTION OF NON-REPETITIVE TASKS, THEIR DURATION, AND TIMING OF BREAKS - TOTAL DURATION

	supply	10		1,0
	cleaning			
	other	10		

Total duration of non-repetitive work per shift (in minutes)	20
Breaks (average): total duration per shift (in minutes): including meal break only if included in the shift	20
Number of breaks (including meal break) lasting at least 8 minutes	3

FIGURE 12.14 Quick Assessment for biomechanical overload of the upper limbs: estimation of the net duration of repetitive work and pauses.

ACCEPTABLE CONDITIONS
If all conditions are described and replies are all "Yes", the risk level is acceptable for repetitive work and it is not necessary to continue the risk evaluation
NB. Please answer all questions by placing an "X" only in the blank spaces

Are one or both upper limbs used less than 50% of the total duration of the repetitive task(s)?	No	X	Yes	
Are both elbows held below shoulder level almost 90% of the total duration of the repetitive task(s)?	No	X	Yes	
Is moderate or no force required (perceived effort = max 3 or 4 on CR-10 Borg scale) by the operator for no more than 1 hour during the repetitive task(s) and are there are no force peaks (perceived effort = 5 or more on CR-10 Borg scale)?	No	X	Yes	
Are there breaks (including meal break) lasting at least 8 minutes every 2 hours and is the repetitive task performed less than 8 hours a day?	No		Yes	X

CRITICAL CONDITIONS
If at least one of the following conditions is present (YES), risk must be considered as CRITICAL and task re-design is URGENTLY REQUIRED.
NB. Please answer all the questions by placing an "X" only in the blank spaces

Are technical actions performed with a single limb so fast that they cannot be counted by simple direct observation?	No	X	Yes	
Are one or both arms used to perform the task with elbow(s) at shoulder level for half or more than the total repetitive working time?	No	X	Yes	
Is a "pinch" grip (or any type of grasp using the finger tips) held for more than 80% of the repetitive working time?	No	X	Yes	
Is peak force applied (perceived effort = 5 or more on the CR-10 Borg scale) for 10% or more of the total repetitive working time?	No	X	Yes	
Is there only one break (including meal break) in a shift of 6-8 hours, or does the total repetitive working time exceed 8 hours in the shift?	No	X	Yes	

FIGURE 12.15 Quick Assessment for biomechanical overload of the upper limbs: check for the presence of acceptable or critical conditions.

Are there other risk factors to be considered when neither critical conditions nor acceptable conditions are present?					
Frequency					
High frequency technical actions performed with the dominant hand					
Slow (no more than 1 action every 2 seconds)	No	X		Yes	
Medium (no more than 1 action per second) or holding an object in the hands most of the time	No			Yes	X
High (more than 1 action per second): difficult to count actions	No	X		Yes	
Shoulder — Are the arms used with the elbow at shoulder level from one third to half of the total repetitive working time?	No			Yes	
Hand — Is a "pinch" grip (or any kind of grasp using the finger tips) used from half to 80% of the repetitive working time?	No			Yes	X
Use of force					
Is peak force (perceived effort = 5 or more on the CR-10 Borg scale) applied from 1% to 9 % of the time?	No	X		Yes	
Is moderate force (perceived effort = max 3 or 4 on the CR-10 Borg scale) required by the operator?	No			Yes	X
indicate the fraction of time (1/3, 2/3, 3/3 of the shift) during which moderate force is used			Duration of moderate	2/3 of time	

FIGURE 12.16 Quick Assessment for biomechanical overload of the upper limbs: risk analysis in the absence of acceptable or critical conditions.

B1	BIOMECHANICAL OVERLOAD OF UPPER LIMBS IN REPETITIVE TASKS	
	SUMMARY OF PRE-ASSESSMENT AND INTERVENTION PRIORITIES	It is necessary to conduct a risk assessment. Intervention is urgent.

FIGURE 12.17 Quick Assessment for biomechanical overload of the upper limbs: Final evaluation with corrective actions in order of priority.

Additional ORGANISATIONAL AND ENVIROMENTAL risk factors to be considered				
Is the working environment unsuitable for manual lifting and carrying?				
There are extreme (low or high) temperatures	No	X	Yes	
Floors are slippery, uneven or unstable	No		Yes	X
There is insufficient space for lifting and carrying	No	X	Yes	
Are the objects unsuitable for manual lifting and carrying?				
The size of the object reduces the operator's view and hinders movement	No		Yes	X
The centre of gravity of the load is not stable (e.g.: liquids, loose items inside a container)	No		Yes	X
The object has sharp edges, rough surfaces or protrusions	No	X	Yes	
Contact surfaces are too cold or too hot	No	X	Yes	
Does the work involve manual lifting or carrying for more than 8 hours a day?	No	X	Yes	

FIGURE 12.18 Quick Assessment for manual load lifting: preliminary factor analysis for the object to be lifted and the working environment.

CRITICAL CONDITIONS					
If only one of the following conditions is present (YES), the risk must be considered high and the task must be immediately re-designed.					
Task lay-out and frequency					
VERTICAL LOCATION	The hand location at the beginning/end of the lift is higher than 175 cm or lower than 0cm	No	x	**Yes**	
VERTICAL DISPLACEMENT	The vertical distance between the origin and the destination of the lifted object is more than 175cm	No	x	**Yes**	
HORIZONTAL DISTANCE	The horizontal distance between the body and load is greater than full arm reach	No	x	**Yes**	
ASYMMETRY	Extreme body twisting without moving the feet	No	x	**Yes**	
FREQUENCY	equal to or higher than 15 times/min with SHORT DURATION (MAX 60 min)	No	x	**Yes**	
	equal to or higher than 12 times/min with MEDIUM DURATION (MAX 120 min)	No	x	**Yes**	
	equal to or higher than 8 times/min with LONG DURATION (OVER 120 min)	No	x	**Yes**	
Loads exceed the following limits					
men (18-45 years)	**25 KG**	No	x	**Yes**	
women (18-45 years)	**20 KG**	No	x	**Yes**	
men (<18 or >45 years)	**20 KG**	No	x	**Yes**	
women (<18 or >45 years)	**15 KG**	No	x	**Yes**	

ACCEPTABLE CONDITIONS				
If NO LOADS >10 KG and all the following conditions are present, and if all replies are "YES" (lifting with both hands) in every weight category (<10KG), the risk level is acceptable for manual load lifting. However, **additional factors must also be checked (see above). NB. Please place an "X" only in white boxes.**				
Loads weigh between 3 and 5 kg		**No**		Yes	x
3 to 5 kg	No asymmetry (e.g. body rotation, trunk twisting)	No	x	Yes	
	Load is held close to the body	No		Yes	x
	Load vertical displacement is between hips and shoulders	No		Yes	x
	Maximum frequency: less than 5 lifts per minute	No	x	Yes	
Loads weigh between 5 and 10 kg		**No**		Yes	x
5 to 10 kg	No asymmetry (e.g. body rotation, trunk twisting)	**No**	x	Yes	
	Load is held close to the body	**No**		Yes	x
	Load vertical displacement is between hips and shoulders	**No**		Yes	x
	Maximum frequency: less than 5 lifts per minute	**No**	x	Yes	
Loads weigh more than 10 kg		No		**Yes**	x

FIGURE 12.19 Quick Assessment for manual load lifting: check for the presence of acceptable or critical conditions.

Characteristics and frequency of certain loads (over 10kg)					
Loads weigh between 10 and 15 kg		No		**Yes**	x
10.5 to 15 kg	No asymmetry (e.g. body rotation, trunk twisting)	**No**		Yes	
	Load is held close to the body	**No**	x	Yes	
	Load vertical displacement is between hips and shoulders	**No**	x	Yes	
	Maximum frequency: less than 1 lift every 5 minutes	**No**	x	Yes	
Loads weigh between 15 and 25 kg		No		**Yes**	x
15.51 to 25 kg	No asymmetry (e.g. body rotation, trunk twisting)	**No**		Yes	
	Load is held close to the body	**No**	x	Yes	
	Load vertical displacement is between hips and shoulders	**No**	x	Yes	
	Maximum frequency: less than 1 lift every 5 minutes	**No**	x	Yes	

FIGURE 12.20 Quick Assessment for manual load lifting: risk analysis for loads weighing more than 10kg.

Conditions of manual carrying					
REPRESENTATIVE PERIOD OF CARRYNG IN A SHIFT (min)	200,0	min			
No. of objects exceeding 3kg carried in a shift	Weight of objects carried	Cumulative mass (kg)	Max. distance (m.):		4m – 10m
100,0	10,0	1000,0			
30,0	25,0	750,0			
		0,0			
		0,0			
Cumulative Mass (total load carried in a shift)) =		1750,0	Does not exceed the limit		
Estimated cumulative mass for each hour =		525,0	Does not exceed the limit		
Estimated cumulative mass for each minute =		8,8	Does not exceed the limit		
Carrying is performed under unfavourable environmental conditions or loads are lifted from/to low levels, e.g. below knee level, or with arms raised above shoulder level			No	Yes	x

FIGURE 12.21 Quick Assessment for manual carrying: comparison between transported cumulative mass and recommended cumulative mass.

BIOMECHANICAL OVERLOAD DUE TO MANUAL PUSHING AND PULLING				
Perceived effort (obtained via worker interviews using the CR-10 Borg scale):			3 – moderato	
Additional organizational and enviromental risk factors to be considered				
Is the working environment unsuitable for pushing or pulling?				
Floors slippery, unstable, uneven, sloping upward or downward or cracked/broken	No		Yes	X
Poor layout makes moving loads awkward	No	X	Yes	
High temperatures in the working area	No		Yes	X
Do the characteristics of the object make it unsuitable for pushing or pulling?				
Object (or trolley, transpallet, etc.) limits the view of the operator or hinders movement	No	X	Yes	
Object is unstable	No		Yes	X
Object (or trolley, transpallet, etc.) has hazardous features, e.g. sharp surfaces, protrusions etc. that may cause injury	No	X	Yes	
Wheels or casters worn, broken or not properly maintained	No		Yes	X
Wheels or casters unsuitable for working conditions	No		Yes	X

FIGURE 12.22 Quick Assessment for manual pushing/pulling: preliminary factor analysis for the object to be handled and the working environment.

12.3.5   Results of the Third and Fourth Parts Concerning the "Quick Assessment" Sections for Awkward Postures

The work sheet on awkward postures must summarize – albeit roughly – all the postures adopted throughout the whole year (Figure 12.25).

12.3.6   Results of the Fifth and Sixth Parts Concerning the "Quick Assessment" Sections for Chemical and Biological Pollutants

The completed work sheets are attached (Figures 12.26 and 12.27).

ACCEPTABLE CONDITIONS				
If all the following conditions are present, and if all replies are "Yes", the risk level is acceptable for pushing-pulling tasks. However, **additional factors must also be checked (see above). NB. Please place an "X" only in the white boxes.**				
Perceived effort (obtained via worker interviews using the CR-10 Borg scale) during pushing-pulling task(s) indicates up to SLIGHT force excertion (perceived effort) (score 2 or less on the Borg CR-10 scale).	No	X	Yes	
Task(s) that include manual pushing and pulling last up to 8 hours a day.	No	X	Yes	
Pushing or pulling force applied to the object between hip and mid-chest level.	No	X	Yes	
Pushing-or-pulling action performed with an upright trunk (not twisted or bent).	No	X	Yes	
Hands held within shoulder width and in front of the body.	No		Yes	X

CRITICAL CONDITIONS				
If just one of conditions indicated below is present (YES), the risk must be considered high and the task must be immediately re-designed.				
Perceived effort (obtained via worker interviews using the CR-10 Borg scale) indicates the use of high peak force (perceived effort) (i.e. a score of 8 or more).	No	X	**Yes**	
Pushing-or-pulling action performed with the trunk significantly bent or twisted.	No	X	**Yes**	
Pushing-or-pulling action performed in a jerky or uncontrolled manner.	No	X	**Yes**	
Hands held either beyond shoulder width or not in front of the body.	No	X	**Yes**	
Hands are held higher than 150 cm or lower than 60 cm.	No	X	**Yes**	
Pushing-or-pulling action combined with vertical force components ("partial lifting").	No	X	**Yes**	
Task(s) that include manual pushing and pulling last more than 8 hours a day.	No	X	**Yes**	

FIGURE 12.23 Quick Assessment for manual pushing/pulling: check for the presence of acceptable or critical conditions.

Summary of manual load handling quick assesment

B2 BIOMECHANICAL OVERLOAD DUE TO LOAD MANUAL LIFTING

SUMMARY OF PRE-ASSESSMENT AND INTERVENTION PRIORITIES	It is necessary to conduct a risk assessment.
	To consider but not urgent.

B3 MECHANICAL OVERLOAD DUE TO MANUAL CARRYING

SUMMARY OF PRE-ASSESSMENT AND INTERVENTION PRIORITIES	It is necessary to conduct a risk assessment.
	To consider but long term.

Summary of additional enviromental factors that are important for MMH

Presence of significative enviromental problems

B4 BIOMECHANICAL OVERLOAD DUE TO MANUAL PULLING AND PUSHING

SUMMARY OF PRE-ASSESSMENT AND INTERVENTION PRIORITIES	It is necessary to conduct a risk assessment.
	To consider but not urgent.

Summary of additional environmental factors that are important for PUSHING and PULLING

Presence of significative enviromental problems

FIGURE 12.24 Quick Assessment for biomechanical overload due to manual handling: final evaluation with corrective actions in order of priority.

12.3.7 RESULTS OF THE SEVENTH PART CONCERNING THE "QUICK ASSESSMENT" AND "PRELIMINARY ANALYSIS" SECTIONS FOR WORK-RELATED STRESS

The workers did not report any major organizational issues or problems with co-workers ("exposure" factor acceptable); certain "sentinel" events or early warning signals are present, such as an increase in time off due to sickness or accident (Figures 12.28 and 12.29).

Trunk posture		
Standing or squatting (not seated)		%time
Nearly always upright		20%
Frequent moderate bending		20%
Frequent twisting		10%
Frequent deep bending		20%
Seated posture		
Works leaning on the back rest		20%
Works in upright position but there is no backrest		
Works mostly bending forward		
Frequent twisting of trunk		10%
Notes:	described duration of trunk posture:	100%

Lower limb postures		
Standing or squatting (not seated)		%time
Standing and able to walk around		50%
Standing in a fixed posture		20%
Kneeling or crouching		
Sitting		%time
Leg room sufficient		30%
Leg room insufficient or very limited		
Leg room non-existent		
Notes:	described duration of lower limb posture:	100%

Use of lower limbs		
		%time
No use of pedals		70%
Lower limbs used to press pedals		30%
Notes:	described duration of lower limb use:	100%

FIGURE 12.25　Quick Assessment for the study of awkward working postures.

12.3.8　SUMMARY OF FINAL RESULTS

Figure 12.30 shows a summary of the final results, with priorities ranked for each risk factor (from 0 to 100%), in relation to the homogeneous group examined here.

12.4　A COMPARISON BETWEEN THE SUMMARY OF FINAL RESULTS FOR THE VARIOUS HOMOGENEOUS GROUPS. CONCLUSIONS

The main purpose of the "simple tool" (**EPMIES-agriERGOCHECKprecultivoENG**) is to avoid complex calculations and automatically prioritize the highly variable dangers and discomfort that farm workers are exposed to; the results of the analysis vary proportionally with the type and level of exposure.

FIGURE 12.26 Quick Assessment for the study of chemical and particulate pollution.

BIOLOGICAL POLLUTANTS POTENTIALLY PRESENT - CRITICALITIES (THIS SECTION MUST BE COMPLETED WHETHER OR NOT BIOLOGICAL POLLUTANTS ARE USED IN THE MANUFACTURING PROCESS)	SPORADIC (1-2 times a month or less)	RARE (no more than 1-2 times a week)	FREQUENT (exposure weekly, but not daily)	VERY FREQUENT (exposure daily)
Presence of centralized air conditioning system with air conditioning unit (AIR TREATMENT UNIT)				
Activities involving water nebulization (spas and wellness centers, showers, etc.)	X			
Activities involving contact with animals, feces and bio-aerosols deriving from same (farms, veterinary and grooming services, pest control, park rangers, etc.)	X			
Activities involving contact with products/substances derived from animals (farms. food industries, slaughterhouses, tanneries, dairies, kitchens, etc.)		X		
Activities involving contact with products/substances derived from plants (agriculture, food industries, paper mills, cosmetics, feed mills, wine cellars, oil presses, carpentry shops,kitchens etc.)				X
Outdoor activities with potential danger of bites by insects, snakes, etc. (example in agriculture)				
Activities involving potential exposure to blood or other biological fluids (health and care professions, child care, research and analytical laboratories, beauticians, tattoo parlors)				
Activities involving the collection, management, treatment, recycling and/or disposal of solid or liquid urban/industrial waste and production of organic fertilizers				
Cleaning and disinfection activities (premises, equipment, materials, etc.) and/or laundering				
Activities involving the use of mineral oils (engineering, etc.)				
Construction activities, animal-free agriculture, involving contact with soil and/or plant- and animal-derived substances			X	
Plant maintenance activities (HVAC, etc.)			X	
Personal care services (kindergartens, nursing homes, barbershops and hairdressers, etc.)				
Activities involving the use of animal and plant metabolites (proteins, enzymes, etc.)	X			
Wholesale/ retail trade excluding contact with plant and animal derived products				
Activities in crowded environments such as schools, gyms etc. (lice, mite allergies ...)				
Transport and storage activities (excluding products of plant and animal origin)				
Manufacturing activities: textile, chemical, pharmaceutical, rubber and plastic industries, hydrocarbon refining or other on signaling.				
NOTES DESCRIBING ANY OTHER AGENTS:				

FIGURE 12.27   Quick Assessment for the study of exposure to biological agents.

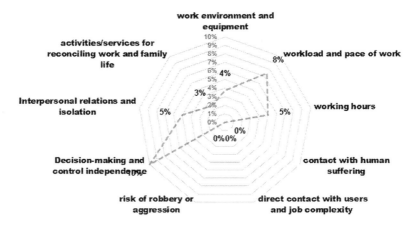

FIGURE 12.28   Quick Assessment of work-related stress: workplace/organizational settings reported by the homogeneous group and graphic depiction (in %) of results for individual risk factors.

	PRESENCE OF THE EVENT LEAVE BLANK IF NONE, MARK WITH AN "X" IF PRESENT	INCREASE IN THE EVENT reported over the last 3 years LEAVE BLANK IF NONE, MARK WITH AN "X" IF	EVENT HIGHER THAN THE COMPANY AVERAGE more frequent than the company average LEAVE BLANK IF NONE.	DESCRIPTIVE NUMERICAL DATA What you have in your possession, enter here some quantitative numeric data specifying the meaning (eg number of events, rate etc.) and the year of reference
Work-related diseases/disorders caused by occupational stress certified by the physician (LEAVE THE BOX BLANK IF NONE)				
Turnover (voluntary resignations)				
Disciplinary actions				
Medical examination requested by the worker		X		
Sick leave		X		
Occupational injuries (not ongoing)		X		

	Hazards						
		HIGH					
X		MEDIUM	**X**				
		LOW					
		ABSENT					
			ACCEPTABLE	LOW	MEDIUM	HIGH	CRITICAL
			X				

Exposure (content and context factors)

FIGURE 12.29 Quick assessment of work-related stress: workplace/organizational settings reported by the homogeneous group (exposure factors) and sentinel (early warning) events for completing a preliminary stress analysis.

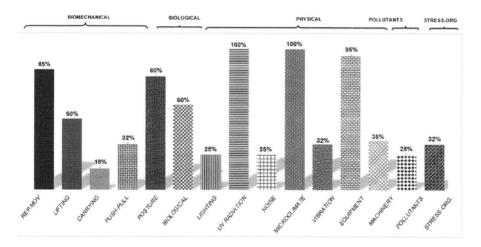

FIGURE 12.30 Summary of results with a ranking of priorities for each risk factor (from 0% to 100%), for the first homogeneous group examined.

Two simple examples are provided (i.e. homogeneous groups 2 and 3), for comparison with the example included in the previous paragraphs of this chapter (homogeneous group 1).

The characteristics of the three homogeneous groups can be summarized as follows:

- Homogeneous group 1: Works 11 months/year and performs a variety of tasks, including driving tractors, pruning and harvesting.
- Homogeneous group 2: Works 3 months/year and only carries out harvesting activities (for over 8 hours a day).
- Homogeneous group 3: Works 3 months/year and only carries out harvesting activities (but for 4 hours a day).

Figure 12.31 summarizes and compares the results in terms of the percentage of hours worked/month (versus a constant 160 hours worked/month) for the three different homogeneous groups. The workers in groups 2 and 3 perform only harvesting activities, group 2 works over 8 hours a day and group 3 works only 4 hours a day.

Figure 12.32 compares the results obtained using **EPMIES-agriERGO CHECKprecultivoENG**: the differences are clear-cut and obvious.

This last example allows us to argue that while complex, an organizational analysis is not only important but essential, even for a preliminary exposure risk analysis. The three examples included in this chapter prove that without a qualitative and quantitative analysis of the tasks performed by the workers, the same risks and the same priorities could be assigned to three different homogeneous groups.

An effort has been made to simplify the organizational analysis through the use of a kind of "universal cultivation" model that includes pre-defined macro-phases and tasks, and various risks are already pre-assigned to tasks. All that remains to be done to complete the organizational study is to assign tasks to each homogeneous group and indicate their duration in percentages.

Another program is also available for defining and determining tasks and risks from scratch (**EPMIES-multiannoERGOCHECKpremapENG**) and can be applied to more specific agricultural cultivations (such as greenhouse crops) and even other industries (e.g. building construction).

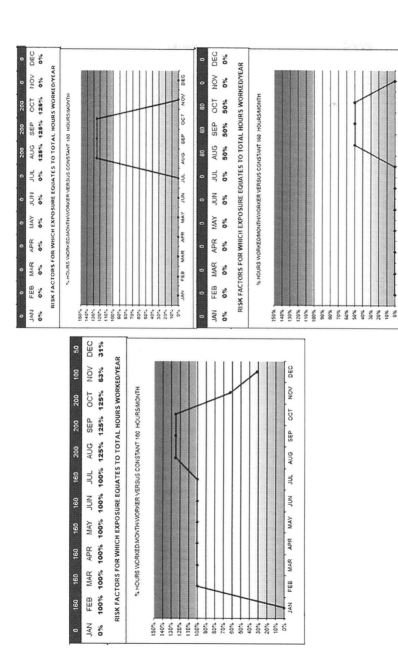

FIGURE 12.31   Summary of results in terms of percentage of hours worked/month (versus constant 160 hours worked/month) for the three homogeneous groups compared here.

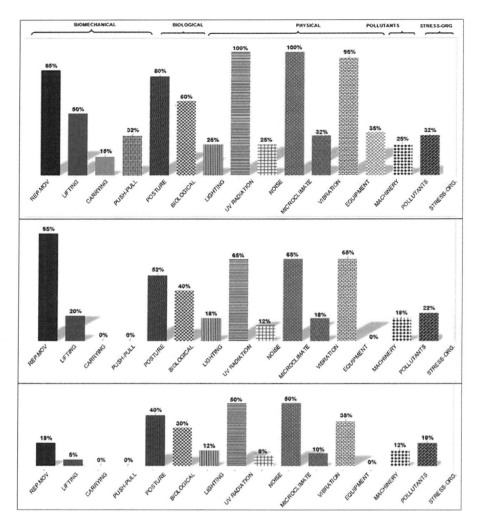

FIGURE 12.32 Summary of results with a ranking of priorities for each of the three different homogeneous groups and for the various risk factor (from 0% to 100%).

13 Conclusions

Daniela Colombini and Enrico Occhipinti
Ergonomics of Posture and Movements
International Ergonomics School (EPM-IES)

These conclusions are, unsurprisingly, brief. Having reached the end of this book, our aims should now be clear, and there should be no need for unnecessary repetition.

Allow us instead to refer to the words of Giulio Maccacaro that appear in the dedication: though dating back to the 1970s, they are still very relevant today.

First of all he argues that: *There is no point in acquiring an abstract snapshot of the production process, what is needed is a real depiction of what each member of the working group experiences as his or her own personal condition.*

Not only for preventative purposes but also for organizational and productive purposes, in order to truly comprehend a working environment: *The traditional approach, based on the "neutrality", "objectivity", "uniqueness" of the production cycle and of the technology and science driving it, is no longer acceptable.*

It is, therefore, also possible to understand the production framework through the direct involvement of the workers, especially groups of workers who are homogeneous in terms of occupational exposure: *Of course, this depiction is not an individualistic view, but rather the result of an evaluation and exploration of the different individualities that contribute, each with their own subjectivity, to constituting the Homogeneous Worker Group and their collective subjectivity. To achieve this, it is necessary to understand how the work of the Homogeneous Worker Group is actually organized and how the group experiences it, together with their working and social background and real working conditions.*

This manual, therefore, seeks to offer methods, criteria, tools and procedures for understanding work and work-related risk, and for prioritizing the implementation of improvements, by specifically analyzing homogeneous groups: subjectivity not at the individual level but at the group level (i.e. collective subjectivity), globality along with simplicity and effectiveness in interpreting the results in order to satisfy real needs.

Thanks again to our mentors: this is not a return to the past but an attempt to look toward the past to find experiences that are not only fundamental for dealing with the present but also the future.

References

ANTLO (Associazione Nazionale Titolari Laboratorio Odontotecnico), 2018. *Panorama mercato odontoiatrico.* www.antlo.it/contenuti/notizie/1936/ANTLO%202018%20(1).pdf.

Ardissone S., 2011. Modelli semplificati di analisi delle sorgenti di rischio e del sovraccarico biomeccanico nel settore artigiano: esperienze applicative nel comparto dei baristi. *La Medicina del Lavoro*; 102, 1:127–137.

ARTEX (Centro per l'artigianato artistico e tradizionale della Toscana), 2008. La ceramica artistica e tradizionale in Italia - Quadro di sintesi, prospettive e fattori di successo. *Atti I Conferenza nazionale della ceramica artistica, Roma 8 ottobre 2008.* www.murmurofart.com/2008/Testo.asp?Progr=3131.

Bakker A.B., Demerouti E., 2007. The job demands resources model: state of the art. *Journal of Managerial Psychology*; 22, 3:309–328.

Bakker A.B., Demerouti E., 2017. Job demands-resources theory: taking stock and looking forward. *Journal of Occupational Health Psychology*; 22:273–285.

Borg G.A.V., 1998. *Borg's Perceived Exertion and Pain Scales.* Human Kinetics, Champaign, IL.

Campanini P., 2014. Analisi degli eventi sentinella: valore aggiunto e metodi. In *Dossier Ambiente n°106. Stress Lavoro-Correlato e Benessere Organizzativo.* Editors C. Bisio e A. Guardavilla. Ambiente e Lavoro, Milano, IT.

Candura F., 1991. *Elementi di tecnologia industriale ad uso dei cultori di Medicina del Lavoro.* Comet Editore, Pavia, IT.

Cannon W.B., 1929. *Bodily Changes in Pain, Hunger, Fear, and Rage.* Appleton and Company, New York.

Cannon W.B., 1932. *Wisdom of the Body.* W.W. Norton & Company, New York.

CDC (Centers for Disease Control and Prevention), 2018. *Prevention guidelines.* https://wonder.cdc.gov/wonder/prevguid/topics.html. (accesso effettuato il 21-11-2018).

CEN (European Committee for Standardization), 2003. EN 1005-2. *Safety of Machinery: Human Physical Performance. Part 2—Manual Handling of Machinery and Component Parts of Machinery.* CEN Management System, Bruxelles, Belgium.

CEN (European Committee for Standardization), 2005. EN-1005-4. *Safety of Machinery – Human Performance – Part 4: Evaluation of Working Postures and Movements in Relation to Machinery.* CEN Management System, Bruxelles, Belgium.

Colombini D., Occhipinti E., 2011. La pre-mappatura dei disagi e dei pericoli professionali e la valutazione e gestione del rischio da sovraccarico biomeccanico: presentazione di uno strumento di analisi semplice e informatizzato (toolkit) e delle sue modalità di utilizzo. *La Medicina del Lavoro*; 102, 1:6–28.

Colombini D., Occhipinti E., 2014. *L'analisi e la gestione del rischio nel lavoro manuale ripetitivo.* Collana Salute e lavoro. Franco Angeli Editore, Milano, IT.

Colombini D., Occhipinti E., 2017. *Risk Analysis and Management of Repetitive Actions – A Guide for Applying the OCRA System.* CRC Press-Taylor and Francis Group, Boca Raton, FL and New York.

Colombini D., Occhipinti E., 2019. *Working Posture Assessment. The TACOs Method.* CRC Press-Taylor and Francis Group, Boca Raton, FL and New York.

Coordinamento Tecnico Interregionale della Prevenzione nei Luoghi di Lavoro, 2012. *Decreto Legislativo 81/2008 e smi. Stress lavoro-correlato: indicazioni per la corretta gestione del rischio e per l'attivita' di vigilanza alla luce della lettera circolare del 18 novembre 2010 del Ministero del lavoro e delle politiche sociali.* http://olympus.uniurb. it/images/stories/regioni-stress-faq-2012.pdf.

Confartigianato Imprese, 2008. Relazione del tavolo di lavoro "Rapporti internazionali"; *Atti I Conferenza nazionale della ceramica artistica, Roma 8 ottobre 2008.* www.murmurofart.com/2008/Testo.asp?Progr=3131.

Confindustria, Confapi, Confartigianato, et al., 2008. *Accordo interconfederale per il recepimento dell'accordo quadro europeo sullo stress lavoro – correlato concluso l'8 ottobre 2004 tra UNICE/UEAPME, CEEP E CES", 9 giugno 2008.* www.servizi.cgil.milano. it/ARCHIVIO/2008/7/20080609_Accordo_StressLavCorrel.pdf.

Di Leone G., Nicoletti S., Monopoli L., Montomoli L., Colombini D., 2011. Utilizzo della scheda di premappatura dei pericoli nel comparto delle ceramiche artistiche. *La Medicina del Lavoro*; 102, 1:43–53.

ETUC, UNICE, UEAPME, CEEP, 2004. *Framework agreement on work related stress.* Bruxelles, 8 ottobre 2004. https://ec.europa.eu/social/search.jsp?advSearch Key=Framework+agreement+on+work+related+stress&mode=advancedSubmit&la ngId=en.

EU-OSHA (European Agency for Safety and Health at Work), 2010. *E-fact n. 53 Risk assessment for biological agents.* https://osha.europa.eu/it/tools-and-publications/ publications/e-facts/efact53.

EUROFOUND, 2017. *Sixth European Working Conditions Survey – Overview Report (2017 Update).* Publications Office of the European Union, Luxembourg.

FIEPET (Federazione Nazionale Esercenti Pubblici e Turistici), 2015. *Osservatorio confesercenti.* www.fiepet.it/imprese-turistiche-aumentano-nel-2%C2%B0-trimestre-2015-ristoranti-e-bar.html

Giambartolomei M., Bolognini P., 2011. Il ciclo tecnologico dell'odontotecnico e i risultati della premappatura dei disagi e dei pericoli. *La Medicina del Lavoro*; 102, 1:54.

HSE (Health and Safety Executive), 2018. *Control of substances hazardous to health (COSHH).* www.hse.gov.uk/coshh/essentials/index.htm.

Jex S.M., Beehr T.A., Roberts C.K., 1992. The meaning of occupational stress items to survey respondents. *Journal of Applied Psychology*; 77, 5:623–628.

Karasek R.A., Theorell T., 1990. *Healthy Work: Stress, Productivity, and the Reconstruction of Working Life.* Basic Books, New York.

Kivimäki M., Virtanen M., Elovainio M., Kouvonen A., Väänänen A., Vahtera J., 2006. Work stress in the etiology of coronary heart disease—a meta-analysis. *Scandinavian Journal of Work, Environment & Health*; 32:431–455.

Kivimäki M., Nyberg S.T., Batty G.D., Fransson E.I., Heikkilä K., Alfredsson, L., Bjorner, J.B., Borritz, M., Burr, H., Casini, A., Clays, E. 2012. Job strain as a risk factor for coronary heart disease: a collaborative meta-analysis of individual participant data. *Lancet*; 380:1491–1497.

ILO (International Labour Office), 2018. *Chemical control banding.* www.ilo.org/legacy/ english/protection/safework/ctrl_banding/.

INAIL (Istituto Nazionale Assicurazione Infortuni sul Lavoro), 2009. *Report dati inail 2009. Bollettino di informazione INAIL ISSN 2035-5645.* www.inail.it/repository/ ContentManagement/node/N670420288/DatiInail%20N7-2010.pdf.

INAIL (Istituto Nazionale Assicurazione Infortuni sul Lavoro), 2011. *Il rischio biologico negli ambienti di lavoro: schede tecnico informative - Ed. 2011. INAIL (IT)* www.inail. it/cs/internet/attivita/prevenzione-e-sicurezza/conoscere-il-rischio/agenti-biologici/ ambienti-di-lavoro.html.

INAIL (Istituto Nazionale Assicurazione Infortuni sul Lavoro), 2018. *Dati Inail 2018; Tavola: IL_DN_IS_AS_ATE_TEM Analisi per attività economica e anno di accadimento.* www.inail.it/cs/internet/attivita/dati-e-statistiche.html.

IOHA (International Occupational Hygiene Association), 2018. *Control banding.* https://ioha.net/control-banding/.

ISO (International Organization for Standardization), 2000. ISO 11226. *Ergonomics— Evaluation of Static Working Postures.* ISO, Geneva, Switzerland.

ISO (International Organization for Standardization), 2003. ISO 11228-1. *Ergonomics: Manual Handling—Lifting and Carrying.* ISO, Geneva, Switzerland.

ISO (International Organization for Standardization), 2007a. ISO 11228-2. *Ergonomics: Manual Handling—Pushing and Pulling.* ISO, Geneva, Switzerland.

ISO (International Organization for Standardization), 2007b. ISO 11228-3. *Ergonomics: Manual Handling—Handling of Low Loads at High Frequency.* ISO, Geneva, Switzerland.

ISO (International Organization for Standardization), 2014. ISO TR 12295. *Ergonomics — Application Document for International Standards on Manual Handling (ISO 11228-1, ISO 11228-2 and ISO 11228-3) and Evaluation of Static Working Postures (ISO 11226).* ISO, Geneva, Switzerland.

Lazarus R.S., 1966. *Psychological Stress and the Coping Process.* McGraw-Hill, New York.

Linton S.J., Kecklund G., Franklin K.A., Leissner L.C., Sivertsen B., Lindberg E., Svensson A.C., Hansson S.O., Sundin Ö., Hetta J., Björkelund, C., 2015. The effect of the work environment on future sleep disturbances: a systematic review. *Sleep Medicine Reviews*; 23:10–19.

Maslach C., Schaufeli W.B., Leiter M.P., 2001. Job burnout. *Annual Review of Psychology*; 52, 1:397–422.

Montomoli L., Coppola G., Sarrini D., Sartorelli P., 2011. Processo della pelle per la produzione di borse: studio organizzativo, identificazione generale dei pericoli, prevalutazione del rischio per il sovraccarico biomeccanico mediante un nuovo strumento di valutazione di semplice applicazione. *La Medicina del Lavoro*; 102, 1:29–42.

Netterstrøm B., Conrad N., Bech P., Fink P., Olsen O., Rugulies R., Stansfeld S., 2008. The relation between work-related psychosocial factors and the development of depression. *Epidemiologic Reviews*; 30, 1:118–132.

Occhipinti E., Colombini D., 2016. A toolkit for the analysis of biomechanical overload and prevention of WMSDs: criteria, procedures and tool selection in a step-by-step approach. *International Journal of Industrial Ergonomics*; 52:18–28.

Rodrigues S.M.L., LeDoux J.E., Sapolsky R.M., 2009. The influence of stress hormones on fear circuitry. *Annual Review of Neuroscience*; 32:289–313.

Sarto D., Caselli U., Giovinazzo R., Guerrera E., Mameli M., 2018. *Il rischio biologico nel mondo del lavoro.* Dossier Ambiente n. 123. Ambiente e Lavoro, Milano, IT.

Selye H., 1936. A syndrome produced by diverse nocuous agents. *Nature*, 138:32.

Selye H., 1974. *Stress Without Distress.* Lippincott, New York.

Siegrist J., Starke D., Chandola T., Godin I., Marmot M., Niedhammer I., Peter, R., 2004. The measurement of effort-reward imbalance at work: European comparisons. *Social Science & Medicine*; 58, 8:1483–1499.

Stansfeld S., Candy B., 2006. Psychosocial work environment and mental health-a meta-analytic review. *Scandinavian Journal of Work, Environment & Health*; 32, 6:443–62.

Waters T.R., Putz-Anderson V., Garg A., Fine L.J., 1993. Revised NIOSH equation for the design and evaluation of manual lifting tasks. *Ergonomics*; 36, 7:749–776.

WHO, 2010. *Healthy workplaces, a model for action: for employers, workers, policymakers and practitioners.* World Health Organization. ISBN 9789241599313. www.who.int/occupational_health/publications/healthy_workplaces_model.pdf.

Index